dr Barbara Pyszczuk

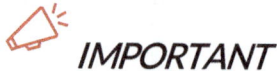

IMPORTANT

You need to have a kidney-friendly meal plan when you have chronic kidney disease (CKD). Watching what you eat, and drink will help you stay healthier. The information in this section is for people who have kidney disease but are not on dialysis.

This information should be used as a basic guide

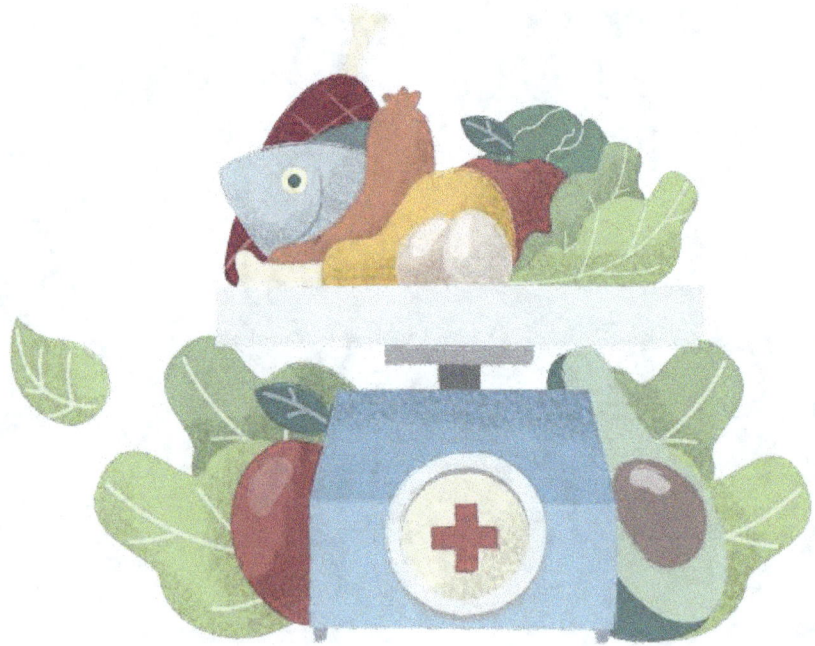

Stages of Chronic Kidney Disease

There are five stages of chronic kidney disease. They are shown in the table below. Your doctor determines your stage of kidney disease, based on the presence of kidney damage and your glomerular filtration rate (GFR), which is a measure of your level of kidney function. Your treatment is based on your stage of kidney disease.

Five Stages of Chronic Kidney Disease		
Stage	Description	Glomerular Filtration Rate (GFR) (ml/min/1,73m2
G1	Kidney damage (e.g., protein in the urine) with normal GFR	90 or above
G2	Kidney damage with mild decrease in GFR	60 to 89
G3a	Moderate decrease in GFR	45 to 59
G3b	Moderate decrease in GFR	30 to 44
G4	Severe reduction in GFR	15 to 29
G5	Kidney failure	Less than 15

*Your GFR number tells your doctor how much kidney function you have. As chronic kidney disease progresses, your GFR number decreases.

Healthy diet basics

With all meal plans, including the kidney-friendly diet, you need to track how much of certain nutrients you take in, such as:

- Calories
- Protein
- Fat
- Carbohydrates

To make sure you are getting the right amounts of these nutrients, you need to eat and drink the right portion sizes

How is a kidney-friendly diet different?

When your kidneys are not working as well as they should, waste and fluid build up in your body. Over time, the waste and extra fluid can cause heart, bone, and other health problems. A kidney-friendly meal plan limits how much of certain minerals and fluid you eat and drink. This can help keep the waste and fluid from building up and causing problems.

How strict your meal plan should be depends on your stage of kidney disease. In the early stages of kidney disease, you may have little or no limits on what you eat and drink. As your kidney disease gets worse, your doctor may recommend that you limit:

- Potassium
- Phosphorus
- Fluids

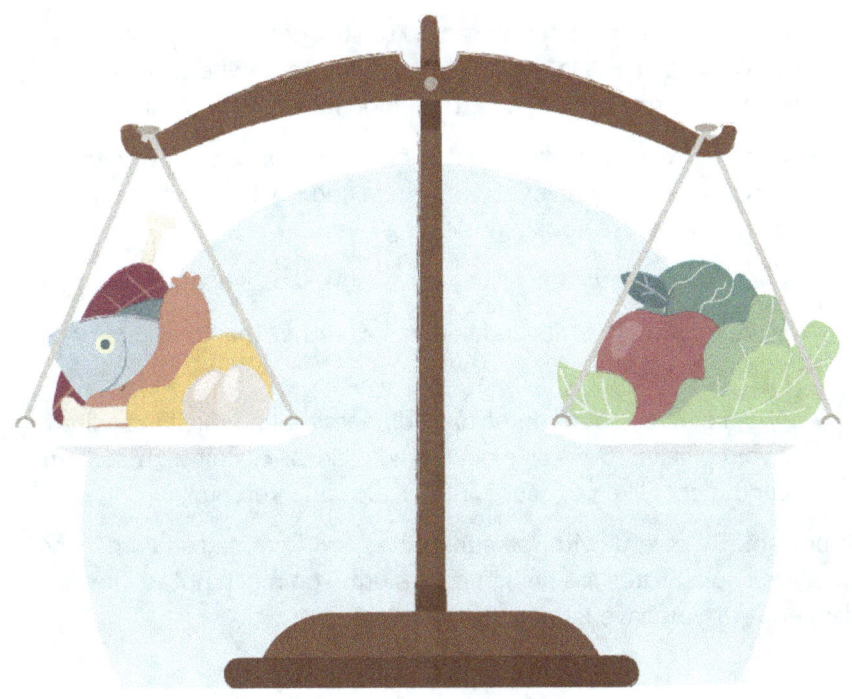

Steps to eating right for chronic kidney disease

1. Choose and prepare foods with less salt

Why?

Sodium (salt) is a mineral found in almost all foods. Too much sodium can make you thirsty, which can lead to swelling and raise your blood pressure. This can damage your kidneys more and make your heart work harder.

One of the best things that you can do to stay healthy, is to limit how much sodium you eat. Do not add salt to your food when cooking or eating. Try cooking with fresh herbs, lemon juice or other salt-free spices.

- Choose fresh or frozen vegetables instead of canned vegetables. If you do use canned vegetables, drain and rinse them to remove extra salt before cooking or eating them.

- Avoid processed meats like ham, bacon, sausage and lunch meats.

- Munch on fresh fruits and vegetables rather than crackers or other salty snacks.

- Avoid canned soups and frozen dinners that are high in sodium. • Avoid pickled foods, like olives and pickles. • Limit high-sodium condiments like soy sauce, BBQ sauce and ketchup.

Important! Be careful with salt substitutes and "reduced sodium" foods. Many salt substitutes are high in potassium. Too much potassium can be dangerous if you have kidney disease.

1 tsp Salt = 2,300mg Sodium

2. Eat the right amount and the right types of protein.

Why?

To help protect your kidneys. When your body uses protein, it produces waste. Your kidneys remove this waste. Eating more protein than you need, may make your kidneys work harder.

Protein can be found in foods from both animals and plants.

Protein and stages of CKD

How much protein do we need to eat to stay healthy? This answer depends on your stage of chronic kidney disease (CKD). It is different for each stage.

CKD stages 1-2

The daily recommended amount of lean protein is the same for people without kidney disease.

CKD stages 3, 4, and 5 (non-dialysis)

For later stage kidney disease, the amount of recommended protein **decreases**. And you should try to get 50-70% of your daily protein from vegetable sources or from fish.

CKD stadium 5 (dializy)

Once you start dialysis, your protein needs **increase**. Dialysis, including hemodialysis and peritoneal dialysis, remove some of your body's blood proteins.

3. Choose foods with the right amount of potassium

Why?

Potassium is a mineral found in almost all foods. Your body needs some potassium to make your muscles work, but too much potassium can be dangerous. When your kidneys are not working well, your potassium level may be too high or too low. Having too much or too little potassium can cause muscle cramps, problems with the way your heart beats and muscle weakness. **Your food and drink choices can help you lower your potassium level, if needed.**

Leaching Potassium from Vegetables

Leaching is the process of pulling potassium out of certain vegetables using water. It's important to remember that leaching will help pull **some** potassium out of high-potassium vegetables, but not all of the potassium. Leaching vegetables does not mean you have free range to eat as much as you want. After leaching potassium from your vegetables, you must still limit how much you eat. Remember to always ask your dietitian or doctor about the amount of leached vegetables that are safe to have in your diet.

How to leach potassium from potatoes and other vegetables:

- Peel the vegetables and slice into 2-inch pieces.
- Rinse the vegetables thoroughly.
- Fill a pot with water and add vegetables (2:1 ratio/water: vegetables).
- Bring the pot of water to a boil, and then drain the water off.
- Fill the pot again with water (2:1 ratio), and boil until soft, but integrity is retained.
- And you're done!

4. Choose foods and drinks with less phosphorus

Why?

To help protect your bones and blood vessels. When you have CKD, phosphorus can build up in your blood. Too much phosphorus in your blood pulls calcium from your bones, making your bones thin, weak, and more likely to break. High levels of phosphorus in your blood can also cause itchy skin, and bone and joint pain.

Phosphorus is added to many foods to help keep the food fresher. Our bodies absorb 100% of what is added. Phosphorus additives can be found in bagged, boxed, canned, or bottled foods. When you have kidney disease, you should avoid or limit foods with these additives. Look on the ingredient list to know if the item has added phosphorus.

- Fresh foods are the best.
- Beware of phosphorus added to packaged foods,
- Always check food labels for "PHOS" to find hidden phosphorus
- Deli meats and some fresh meat and poultry can have added phosphorus.

A quick way to spot added phosphorus is to look for phosphates or "phos" in the ingredient list.

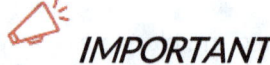 *IMPORTANT*

- *Milk and dairy products are high in phosphorus.*
- *Try dairy substitutes like rice milk that are lower in phosphorus*
  - *Instead of milk → unfortified rice milk*
  - *Instead of ice cream → sorbet*

How a Low-Protein Diet Can Delay Dialysis in Patients With Chronic Kidney Disease

- A low-protein diet (< 0.8 g/kg/d) has been shown to potentially preserve kidney function longer in individuals with chronic kidney disease (CKD).

- Evidence suggests that a low-protein diet consistently reduces intraglomerular pressure, which may help maintain kidney function over the long term.

- Most studies recommend a protein intake ranging from 0.6 to less than 0.8 grams per kilogram per day for managing CKD.

- However, some research indicates that consuming less than 0.6 grams per kilogram per day might further slow CKD progression.

- Therefore, aiming for a protein intake within the range of 0.6 to less than 0.8 grams per kilogram per day is considered the safest and most practical approach, especially if no amino acid or keto acid supplements are used.

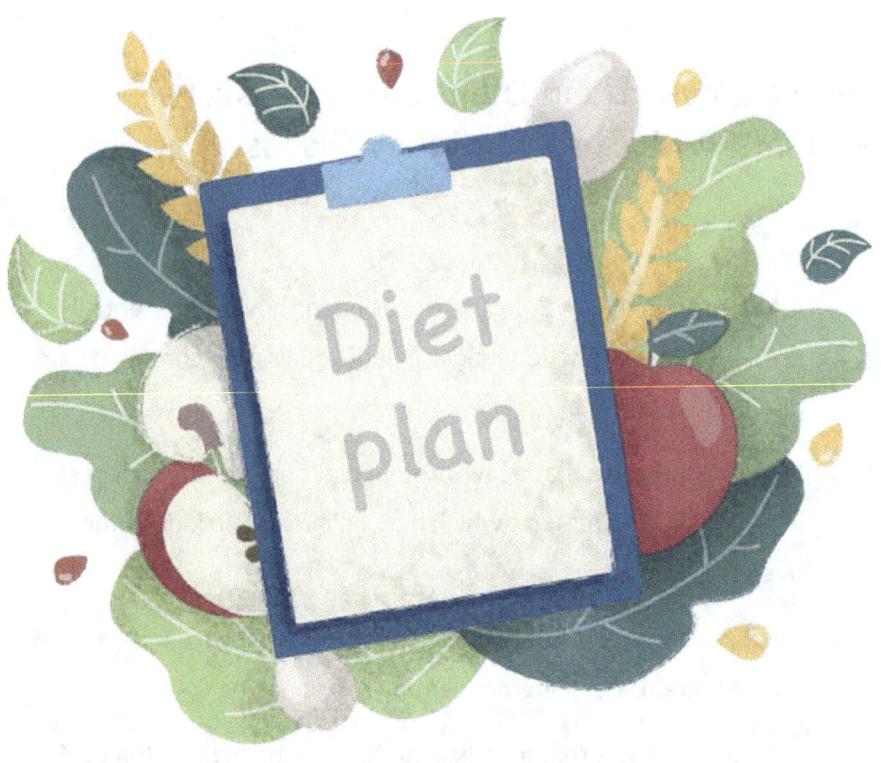

Nutrition is important for proper development and health. The body should be provided with an appropriate amount of food products so that the energy and nutrients contained in them cover the body's needs.

If you don't manage to follow the diet on a given day, don't blame yourself for it and don't make any special restrictions for yourself for the next day. Return normally to the planned plan

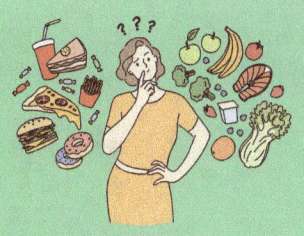

LOW PROTEIN DIET

14 NUTRITION PLAN

dr Barbara Pyszczuk

MEAL SCHEDULE

DAY 1

Energy: 2043 kcal · Protein: 49 g · Fat: 78 g · Carbohydrates: 302 g · Phosphorus: 1046.89 mg · Potassium: 2713.87 mg · Sodium: 1938.38 mg

Diet:5 meals | 2000 kcal | B: 50 g | low protein

Breakfast

Product	Kcal	Weight	Home measure
Rice milk	94	200 g	200 ml
Semolina	173	48 g	4 tbsp
Coconut shreds	119	18 g	3 tbsp
Raspberries	62	120 g	2 handful
Maple syrup	14	5 g	1tsp

Kcal: 462 • P: 9 g • F: 15 g • C: 75 g • P: 249 mg • K: 433 mg • Na: 87 mg

Coconut semolina with fruit

Preparation:

1. Boil milk and add semolina and 2 tablespoons of coconut shavings stir all the time.

2. Transfer to a bowl, add fruit and top with maple syrup. Sprinkle with the remaining roasted coconut shavings.

Second breakfast

Product	Kcal	Weight	Home measure
Light rye bread	75	30 g	1 slice
Mango	54	90 g	2 slice
Turkey ham	33	30 g	2 slice
Lettuce butterhead	8	60 g	2 handful
Lemon juice	5	24 g	4 tbsp
Olive oil	133	15 g	3tsp

Kcal: 308 • P: 11 g • F: 17 g • C: 34 g • P: 159 mg • K: 445 mg • Na: 458 mg

Turkey and mango salad

Preparation:

1. Toast bread in a toaster oven and cut and dice.

2. Dice mango and ham, and tear lettuce into smaller pieces.

3. Mix all ingredients.

4. Pour dressing prepared from lemon juice and olive oil over salad. Sprinkle croutons on top.

Lunch

Product	Kcal	Weight	Home measure
Rice noodles	655	180 g	180g
Onion	23	70 g	small 1 piece
Canola oil	177	20 g	2 tbsp
Garlic	12	8 g	2 clove
Zucchini	42	200 g	medium 0.5 piece
Canned chopped tomatoes	96	300 g	300g
Chickpeas in brine	152	120 g	6 tbsp
Salt	0	1 g	1 pinch
Parsley leaves	9	24 g	2 tbsp

Kcal: 1166 • P: 32 g • F: 26 g • C: 199 g • P: 700 mg • K: 2274 mg • Na: 1455 mg

1 servings:
Kcal: 583 • P: 16 g • F: 13 g • C: 100 g • P: 350 mg • K: 1137 mg • Na: 728 mg

Vegan cureo with pasta 🌙

Multiple servings recipe - 1/2 servings

Preparation:

1. Cook pasta according to the instructions on the package.

2. Peel, chop and fry onion in oil along with the garlic in a large pot.

3. Cut zucchini into cubes.

4. Add canned tomatoes, chickpeas to pan and simmer for 15 minutes.

5. Add some water, if necessary.

6. Finally, add salt, season and sprinkle with parsley .

Snack

Product	Kcal	Weight	Home measure
Hummus	142	60 g	3 tbsp
Light rye bread	150	60 g	2 slice
Radish sprouts	10	24 g	3 tbsp

Kcal: 303 • P: 8 g • F: 12 g • C: 44 g • P: 211 mg • K: 307 mg • Na: 619 mg

Sandwiches with hummus

Preparation:

1. Spread paste on the bread.

2. Decorate sandwiches with sprouts.

Dinner

Product	Kcal	Weight	Home measure
Pepper red	16	60 g	medium 0.5 piece
Carrot	17	50 g	small 1 piece
Canola oil	177	20 g	2 tbsp
Parsley leaves	4	12 g	1 tbsp
White rice	175	50 g	0.5 package

Kcal: 388 • P: 5 g • F: 21 g • C: 48 g • P: 79 mg • K: 392 mg • Na: 47 mg

Vegetable salad with rice

Preparation:

1. Cut peppers and carrots into strips and fry in 1 tablespoon of oil.

2. Cook rice according to the instructions on the package.

3. Put vegetables in a bowl, add chopped parsley, rice, the rest of the oil and mix.

4. Season whole thing to taste.

DAY 2

Energy: 2017 kcal • Protein: 50 g • Fat: 63 g • Carbohydrates: 330 g • Phosphorus: 1038.65 mg • Potassium: 2761.72 mg • Sodium: 1432.06 mg

Diet: 5 meals | 2000 kcal | B: 50 g | low protein

Breakfast

Product	Kcal	Weight	Home measure
Oat flakes	152	40 g	4 tbsp
Coconut yogurt	118	125 g	5 tbsp
Natural yogurt 2%	24	40 g	2 tbsp
Pineapple	108	240 g	3 slice
Coconut shreds	40	6 g	1 tbsp

Kcal: 441 • P: 10 g • F: 16 g • C: 68 g • P: 247 mg • K: 557 mg • Na: 42 mg

Oatmeal with pineapple

Preparation:

1. Pour flakes into a saucepan, water, cook about 5- 6 minutes stirring.

2. To finished oatmeal add remaining ingredients.

Second breakfast

Product	Kcal	Weight	Home measure
Vegetable broth	50	500 g	2 glass
Broccoli	93	300 g	300g
Olive oil	177	20 g	2 tbsp
Almonds flakes	116	20 g	2 tbsp
Garlic	18	12 g	3 clove
Light rye bread	175	70 g	2.3 slice
Basil fresh	2	10 g	1 handful

Kcal: 631 • P: 18 g • F: 35 g • C: 74 g • P: 406 mg • K: 1591 mg • Na: 1950 mg

1 servings:
Kcal: 315 • P: 9 g • F: 17 g • C: 37 g • P: 203 mg • K: 795 mg • Na: 975 mg

Broccoli soup with toast 🌙

Multiple servings recipe - 1/2 servings

Preparation:

1. Add broccoli florets and pressed garlic to boiling vegetable stock.

2. Cook until broccoli is tender.

3. Season to taste,

4. Blend the soup into a cream with 2 tablespoons of olive oil. Sprinkle with roasted almond flakes.
5. Toast the bread in a toaster oven. Mix the remaining olive oil with basil. Spread the oil on the croutons.

Lunch

Product	Kcal	Weight	Home measure
Potatoes	87	150 g	medium 2 piece
Onion	23	70 g	small 1 piece
Canola oil	265	30 g	3 tbsp
Quark half-fat	79	60 g	3 tbsp
Salt	0	1 g	1 pinch
Pepper black	5	2 g	2 pinch
Turmeric ground	6	2 g	1tsp
Wheat white flour	437	120 g	8 tbsp
Rice flour white	366	100 g	10 tbsp
Water	0	150 g	150 ml

Kcal: 1269 • P: 35 g • F: 36 g • C: 200 g • P: 450 mg • K: 1045 mg • Na: 438 mg

1 servings:
Kcal: 634 • P: 17 g • F: 18 g • C: 100 g • P: 225 mg • K: 522 mg • Na: 219 mg

Homemade dumplings 🌙

Multiple servings recipe - 1/2 servings

Preparation:

1. Peel and cut potatoes into smaller pieces. Transfer to a pot of water and cook until tender, about 20-25 minutes.

2. At this time, cut onions into small cubes and fry them in oil until browned.

3. Put cottage cheese into a bowl and mash it with a fork. Add the fried onions and mix.

4. Drain the boiled potatoes and add to bowl. Mash with a pestle until the ingredients are thoroughly combined.

5. Add spices, mix and set aside.

6. In a separate bowl, add flour (230 g) oil and salt, and finally hot water. Mix with a spoon and then knead dough with your hands.

7. Form a ball and divide it into 4 parts.

8. Dust the dough with the remaining flour. Roll it out, cut out circles with a glass.

9. Put 2 teaspoons of stuffing each on the dough pieces and seal the dumplings.

10. Drop half of dumplings into a pot of boiling water. Cook about 2 minutes from the moment they float to surface of the water.

Snack

Product	Kcal	Weight	Home measure
Coconut yogurt	75	80 g	0.5 packaging
Natural yogurt 2%	37	60 g	3 tbsp
Cocoa powder	11	5 g	1tsp
Blueberries	29	50 g	1 handful
Nectarine	48	110 g	small 1 piece
Raspberries	31	60 g	1 handful

Kcal: 231 • P: 7 g • F: 8 g • C: 38 g • P: 162 mg • K: 546 mg • Na: 46 mg

Yogurt with fruit

Preparation:

1. Mix yogurt with remaining ingredients.

Dinner

Product	Kcal	Weight	Home measure
Rice noodles	218	60 g	60g
Raspberries	62	120 g	2 handful
Natural yogurt 2%	37	60 g	3 tbsp
Honey	73	24 g	2tsp
Cinnamon ground	5	2 g	0.5 tsp

Kcal: 395 • P: 8 g • F: 2 g • C: 88 g • P: 202 mg • K: 340 mg • Na: 149 mg

Pasta with raspberry sauce

Preparation:

1. Cook pasta according to the instructions on the package.

2. Crush raspberries, add yogurt and honey, mix.

3. Pour sauce over pasta, sprinkle with cinnamon.

DAY 3

Energy: 1959 kcal • Protein: 48 g • Fat: 88 g • Carbohydrates: 264 g • Phosphorus: 1087.03 mg • Potassium: 2574.82 mg • Sodium: 3906.37 mg

Diet:5 meals | 2000 kcal | B: 50 g | low protein

Breakfast

Product	Kcal	Weight	Home measure
Cabbage chinese pe-tsai	16	100 g	100g
Red tomato	11	60 g	medium 0.5 piece
Onion	12	35 g	small 0.5 piece
Pepper red	10	38 g	small 0.5 piece
Corn sweet canned	19	30 g	2 tbsp
Olive oil	88	10 g	1 tbsp
Lemon juice	1	6 g	1 tbsp
Sweet pepper spice	3	1 g	1 pinch
Salt	0	1 g	1 pinch
Pepper black	3	1 g	1 pinch
Light rye bread	150	60 g	2 slice
Butter	100	14 g	2tsp
Turkey ham	17	15 g	1 slice

Kcal: 429 • P: 10 g • F: 24 g • C: 50 g • P: 205 mg • K: 721 mg • Na: 952 mg

Sandwiches and salad of Chinese cabbage

Preparation:

1. Chop vegetables and mix with olive oil, lemon juice and spices.

2. Spread bread with butter, add ham.

3. Sandwich eat with salad.

Second breakfast

Product	Kcal	Weight	Home measure
Coconut yogurt	150	160 g	1 packaging
Raspberries	31	60 g	1 handful
Coconut shreds	79	12 g	2 tbsp
Walnuts	52	8 g	2 piece

Kcal: 313 • P: 4 g • F: 25 g • C: 22 g • P: 70 mg • K: 191 mg • Na: 18 mg

Coconut yogurt with raspberries

Preparation:

1. Mix yogurt with all ingredients.

Lunch

Product	Kcal	Weight	Home measure
Corn pasta	357	100 g	100g
Tomatoes cherry	11	60 g	3 piece
Basil pesto	149	40 g	2 tbsp
Arugula	4	20 g	1 handful
Parmesan cheese	63	16 g	2 tbsp

Kcal: 583 • P: 16 g • F: 21 g • C: 86 g • P: 429 mg • K: 603 mg • Na: 611 mg

Pasta with pesto and tomatoes

Preparation:

1. Cook pasta according to the instructions on the package.

2. Cut tomatoes in half.

3. Mix pesto with warm pasta and tomatoes.

4. Sprinkle with grated cheese and add arugula.

Snack

Product	Kcal	Weight	Home measure
Strawberries	22	70 g	1 handful
Raspberries	31	60 g	1 handful
Blueberries	29	50 g	1 handful
Gelatin desserts dry mix	164	43 g	0.5 packaging
Natural yogurt 2%	12	20 g	1 tbsp

Kcal: 258 • P: 6 g • F: 1 g • C: 60 g • P: 125 mg • K: 279 mg • Na: 215 mg

Fruit in jelly

Preparation:

1. Prepare jelly according to the instructions on package.

2. Wash the fruits and pour over jelly. Put in refrigerator to let jelly set.

3. Add yogurt on top of dessert.

Dinner

Product	Kcal	Weight	Home measure
Butter	100	14 g	2tsp
Spinach	11	75 g	3 handful
Egg	70	50 g	1 medium piece
Light rye bread	150	60 g	2 slice
Red tomato	31	170 g	1 piece
Pickled cucumber	14	130 g	2 medium piece

Kcal: 376 • P: 12 g • F: 18 g • C: 46 g • P: 258 mg • K: 781 mg • Na: 2111 mg

Scrambled eggs with spinach

Preparation:

1. Heat half of butter in a pan, throw in spinach and blanch.

2. Whisk egg with salt and pepper in a separate dish. Pour into skillet.

3. Stir constantly until the egg is set.

4. Spread bread with butter and add tomato slices and pickled cucumber.

DAY 4

Energy: 1936 kcal • Protein: 51 g • Fat: 76 g • Carbohydrates: 284 g • Phosphorus: 923.91 mg • Potassium: 3672.52 mg • Sodium: 2490.79 mg

Diet: 5 meals | 2000 kcal | B: 50 g | low protein

Breakfast

Product	Kcal	Weight	Home measure
Lettuce butterhead	1	10 g	2 leaf
Apple	36	70 g	0.5 piece medium
Leek	31	50 g	1 piece
Dill fresh	2	5 g	1tsp
Orange	50	80 g	small 0.5 piece
Olive oil	44	5 g	1tsp
Light rye bread	150	60 g	2 slice
Butter	100	14 g	2tsp
Italian style cheese Capri (Sierpc)	56	30 g	3tsp

Kcal: 472 • P: 8 g • F: 22 g • C: 65 g • P: 128 mg • K: 485 mg • Na: 439 mg

Sandwiches and apple salad

Preparation:

1. wash and chop the lettuce.

2. Grate apple on a coarse grater.

3. Chop leek and dill finely.

4. Mix the vegetables with the apple. Add orange juice and oil.

5. Season to taste and set aside in the refrigerator for 30 minutes.

6. Prepare croutons from bread in a toaster oven or oven. Then spread with butter and add capri cheese.

7. Eat salad with croutons.

Second breakfast

Product	Kcal	Weight	Home measure
Light rye bread	150	60 g	2 slice
Butter	50	7 g	1tsp
Italian style cheese Capri (Sierpc)	38	20 g	2tsp
Red tomato	22	120 g	medium 1 piece
Onions green spring or scallions	5	15 g	medium 1 piece
Olive oil	44	5 g	1tsp
Salt	0	1 g	1 pinch
Pepper black	3	1 g	1 pinch

Kcal: 311 • P: 6 g • F: 15 g • C: 42 g • P: 113 mg • K: 441 mg • Na: 799 mg

Italian sandwiches

Preparation:

1. Spread butter on sandwiches, add sliced Capri cheese.

2. Cut tomato into eights, mix with sliced onion. Drizzle the whole thing with olive oil, season.

Lunch

Product	Kcal	Weight	Home measure
Olive oil	44	5 g	1tsp
Shallot	14	20 g	2 tbsp
Garlic	7	5 g	1.3 clove
Peppers hot red chili	2	5 g	1 piece
Ginger root	2	2 g	1tsp
Button mushrooms	11	50 g	small 5 piece
Curry paste	5	5 g	0.5 tsp
Coriander leaves	1	5 g	5 g
Zucchini	17	80 g	8 slice
Coconut milk canned 19%	94	50 g	5 tbsp
Water	0	200 g	200 ml
Broccoli	16	50 g	50g
Green beans frozen	17	50 g	1 handful
Chickpeas canned	106	120 g	6 tbsp
Spinach	4	25 g	1 handful
Lime juice	2	9 g	3tsp
Jasmine rice	174	50 g	5 tbsp

Kcal: 515 • P: 18 g • F: 18 g • C: 77 g • P: 305 mg • K: 1282 mg • Na: 339 mg

Vegetarian curry with chickpeas

Preparation:

1. Pour oil into large pot or wok, add sliced shallots, garlic, chili, ginger and simmer for about 3 minutes.

2. Add chopped vegetables, first mushrooms, after another 3 minutes add curry paste, a few sprigs of coriander and zucchini.

3. Simmer for about 4 minutes.

4. Pour in milk and 200 ml of water.

5. Cook for 5 minutes, add broccoli, beans and chickpeas.

6. After 5-6 minutes, add spinach and season with lime juice.

7. Serve with cooked rice and rest of coriander.

Snack

Product	Kcal	Weight	Home measure
Water	0	250 g	1 glass
Pineapple	50	110 g	1 serving
Lemon juice	7	30 g	5 tbsp
Ginger root	3	4 g	2 slice
Linseed	27	5 g	1tsp
Parsley leaves	9	24 g	2 tbsp
Biscuits	171	45 g	large 5 piece

Kcal: 265 • P: 7 g • F: 5 g • C: 52 g • P: 138 mg • K: 409 mg • Na: 88 mg

Smoothie with pineapple and parsley

Preparation:

1. Blend all ingredients, adding water as needed. 2. Eat biscuits.

Dinner

Product	Kcal	Weight	Home measure
Beets cooked	106	240 g	2 piece
Arugula	4	20 g	1 handful
Ricotta cheese	90	60 g	3 tbsp
Lemon juice	3	12 g	2 tbsp
Olive oil	88	10 g	1 tbsp
Salt	0	1 g	1 pinch
Pepper black	5	2 g	2 pinch
Basil fresh	2	10 g	1 handful
Light rye bread	75	30 g	1 slice

Kcal: 373 • P: 11 g • F: 17 g • C: 49 g • P: 241 mg • K: 1056 mg • Na: 826 mg

Beet carpaccio on arugula and cottage cheese

Preparation:

1. Cut beets into thin slices.

2 Arrange a handful of arugula in the center of the plate, and overlap the beet slices all around. Add ricotta cheese.

3. Mix lemon juice well with olive oil, salt and pepper. Pour the dressing over the salad. Decorate whole thing with basil.

4. Serve with bread toasted in the toaster or oven.

DAY 5

Energy: 1613 kcal • Protein: 52 g • Fat: 54 g • Carbohydrates: 244 g • Phosphorus: 866.89 mg • Potassium: 2375.02 mg • Sodium: 2035.55 mg

Diet:5 meals | 2000 kcal | B: 50 g | low protein

Breakfast

Product	Kcal	Weight	Home measure
Millet	170	45 g	3 tbsp
Apple	73	140 g	medium 1 piece
Water	0	15 g	1 tbsp
Raisins seedless	27	9 g	1 tbsp
Almonds	58	10 g	10 piece
Lemon juice	1	6 g	2tsp
Maple syrup	27	10 g	1 tbsp

Kcal: 356 • P: 8 g • F: 7 g • C: 69 g • P: 201 mg • K: 406 mg • Na: 7 mg

Sweet millet groats with apple

Preparation:

1. Rinse millet in cold water and cook it according to the recipe on the package.

2. Peel and slice apple and stew in a pot with a tablespoon of water for about 10 minutes.

3. Add raisins, chopped almonds and drizzle with

lemon
juice.

4. Add millet and mix with the honey.

Second breakfast

Product	Kcal	Weight	Home measure
Wheat roll	218	80 g	1 piece
Butter	50	7 g	1tsp
Ricotta cheese	30	20 g	1 tbsp
Strawberry jam low-sugar	15	10 g	1tsp

Kcal: 314 • P: 8 g • F: 9 g • C: 51 g • P: 92 mg • K: 141 mg • Na: 326 mg

Wheat bun with cottage cheese and jam

Preparation:

1. Cut roll in half, spread with butter, cheese and jam.

Lunch

Product	Kcal	Weight	Home measure
Carrot	10	30 g	medium 0.5 piece
Parsley root	14	40 g	0.5 piece
Celery	3	23 g	0.5 piece
Broth	74	150 g	150 ml
Pepper black	3	1 g	1 pinch
Salt	0	1 g	1 pinch
Dill fresh	4	10 g	2tsp
Millet	113	30 g	2 tbsp
Cauliflower	26	105 g	7 floret
Allspice spice	3	1 g	1 grain
Bay leaf	3	1 g	1 leaf
Olive oil	44	5 g	1tsp

Kcal: 297 • P: 16 g • F: 11 g • C: 37 g • P: 186 mg • K: 862 mg • Na: 1091 mg

Dill soup with cauliflower and millet

Preparation:

1. Peel, wash and dice carrots, parsley and celery.

2. Pour in broth, add water, bay leaves and allspice.

3. Boil under the lid for 15 minutes. Add cauliflower florets and cook for 5 minutes together.

4. Add millet and cook until tender.

5. Towards the end of cooking add olive oil and chopped dill.

6. Season soup to taste.

Snack

Product	Kcal	Weight	Home measure
Light rye bread	150	60 g	2 slice
Italian style cheese Capri (Sierpc)	75	40 g	4tsp
Avocado	24	15 g	1 slice
Lettuce butterhead	4	30 g	1 handful

Kcal: 253 • P: 8 g • F: 9 g • C: 38 g • P: 93 mg • K: 244 mg • Na: 444 mg

Capri cheese and lettuce sandwiches

Preparation:

1. Spread the sandwiches with capri cheese.

2. Add lettuce and sliced avocado.

Dinner

Product	Kcal	Weight	Home measure
Corn pasta	179	50 g	50g
Avocado	112	70 g	0.5 piece
Lettuce butterhead	8	60 g	2 handful
Radish	5	30 g	2 piece
Mozzarella cheese	90	30 g	2 slice

Kcal: 393 • P: 13 g • F: 18 g • C: 49 g • P: 295 mg • K: 722 mg • Na: 167 mg

Salad with noodles and avocado

Preparation:

1. Cook pasta according to instructions on the package.

2. Chop vegetables and mozzarella.

3. Mix all ingredients.

4. Season.

DAY 6

Energy: 2189 kcal • Protein: 47 g • Fat: 91 g • Carbohydrates: 315 g • Phosphorus: 1043.43 mg • Potassium: 3558.13 mg • Sodium: 1588.12 mg

Diet:5 meals | 2000 kcal | B: 50 g | low protein

Breakfast

Product	Kcal	Weight	Home measure
White rice	210	60 g	4 tbsp
Pear	107	160 g	small 1 piece
Ginger ground	7	2 g	1tsp
Cinnamon ground	2	1 g	1 pinch
Turmeric ground	3	1 g	1 pinch
Coconut shreds	119	18 g	3 tbsp

Kcal: 448 • P: 6 g • F: 12 g • C: 80 g • P: 109 mg • K: 391 mg • Na: 13 mg

Spiced rice with pear

Preparation:

1. Cook rice according to the instructions on the package. 2. Cut fruit into cubes. Mix with spices.

3. Put rice on a plate add pear and coconut shavings.

Second breakfast

Product	Kcal	Weight	Home measure
Ricotta cheese	150	100 g	5 tbsp
Natural yogurt 2%	24	40 g	2 tbsp
Raspberries	31	60 g	1 handful
Blueberries	29	50 g	1 handful
Biscuits	68	18 g	large 2 piece

Kcal: 302 • P: 12 g • F: 12 g • C: 37 g • P: 257 mg • K: 448 mg • Na: 163 mg

Ricotta cheese with raspberries

Preparation:

1. Mix cheese with yogurt and fruit.

2. Eat with biscotti.

Lunch

Product	Kcal	Weight	Home measure
Corn pasta	357	100 g	100g
Tomatoes cherry	11	60 g	3 piece
Basil pesto	149	40 g	2 tbsp
Arugula	4	20 g	1 handful
Parmesan cheese	63	16 g	2 tbsp

Kcal: 583 • P: 16 g • F: 21 g • C: 86 g • P: 429 mg • K: 603 mg • Na: 611 mg

Pasta with pesto and tomatoes

Preparation:

1. Cook pasta according to the instructions on the package.

2. Cut tomatoes in half.

3. Mix pesto with warm pasta and tomatoes.

4. Sprinkle with grated cheese and add arugula.

Snack

Product	Kcal	Weight	Home measure
Coconut milk canned light 6%	80	120 g	0.5 glass
Coconut cream	61	10 g	1tsp
Avocado	112	70 g	0.5 piece
Orange	101	160 g	small 1 piece
Banana	89	100 g	small 1 piece
Ginger root	2	2 g	1tsp

Kcal: 444 • P: 7 g • F: 24 g • C: 57 g • P: 94 mg • K: 1281 mg • Na: 41 mg

Green smoothies

Preparation:
1. Blend the ingredients.

Dinner

Product	Kcal	Weight	Home measure
Avocado	112	70 g	0.5 piece
Lemon juice	1	6 g	1 tbsp
Olive oil	88	10 g	1 tbsp
Salt	0	1 g	1 pinch
Pepper black	3	1 g	1 pinch
Light rye bread	150	60 g	2 slice
Red tomato	11	60 g	medium 0.5 piece
Kiwi	46	75 g	1 piece

Kcal: 411 • P: 5 g • F: 22 g • C: 55 g • P: 153 mg • K: 835 mg • Na: 760 mg

Toast with avocado, kiwi

Preparation:

1. Mash avocado with a fork. Add lemon juice, olive oil, salt and pepper, mix.

2. Spread the bread slices with paste, add tomato slices.

3. Eat fruit separately.

DAY 7

Energy: 1850 kcal • Protein: 52 g • Fat: 90 g • Carbohydrates: 224 g • Phosphorus: 722.55 mg • Potassium: 2512.65 mg • Sodium: 1513.84 mg

Diet:5 meals | 2000 kcal | B: 50 g | low protein

Breakfast

Product	Kcal	Weight	Home measure
Buttery croissant (Lidl)	322	100 g	1 piece
Butter	50	7 g	1tsp
Strawberry jam low-sugar	76	50 g	5tsp

Kcal: 448 • P: 9 g • F: 11 g • C: 77 g • P: 5 mg • K: 31 mg • Na: 1 mg

Buttery croissant with jam

Preparation:

1. Cut the roll in half. Spread with butter and jam.

Second breakfast

Product	Kcal	Weight	Home measure
Coconut yogurt	150	160 g	1 packaging
Raspberries	31	60 g	1 handful
Coconut shreds	79	12 g	2 tbsp
Walnuts	52	8 g	2 piece

Kcal: 313 • P: 4 g • F: 25 g • C: 22 g • P: 70 mg • K: 191 mg • Na: 18 mg

Coconut yogurt with raspberries

Preparation:

1. Mix yogurt with all ingredients.

Lunch

Product	Kcal	Weight	Home measure
Atlantic salmon	166	80 g	80g
Lemon juice	1	6 g	1 tbsp
Sesame	29	5 g	1tsp
Potatoes	157	270 g	large
			3. piece
Olive oil	88	10 g	1 tbsp
Dill fresh	4	10 g	1 tbsp
Apple	36	70 g	medium
			0.5 piece
Carrot	17	50 g	small
			1 piece
Horseraddish grated	4	4 g	1tsp
Canola oil	88	10 g	1 tbsp
Salt	0	1 g	1 pinch
Pepper black	3	1 g	1 pinch

Kcal: 594 • P: 25 g • F: 34 g • C: 50 g • P: 360 mg • K: 1767 mg • Na: 523 mg

Grilled salmon with potatoes

Preparation:

1. Drizzle the salmon with lemon juice, coat with sesame seeds and grill for 3-4 minutes.

2. Doil the potatoes, then drizzle with olive oil and sprinkle with chopped dill.

3. Grate the apple and carrot on a small-mesh grater, mix with the chan and oil. Season.

4. Serve salmon with potatoes and carrot salad.

Snack

Product	Kcal	Weight	Home measure
Hummus	142	60 g	3 tbsp
Light rye bread	150	60 g	2 slice
Radish sprouts	10	24 g	3 tbsp

Kcal: 303 • P: 8 g • F: 12 g • C: 44 g • P: 211 mg • K: 307 mg • Na: 619 mg

Sandwiches with hummus

Preparation:

1. Spread paste on the bread.

2. Decorate sandwiches with sprouts.

Dinner

Product	Kcal	Weight	Home measure
Wheat-rye bread	135	60 g	2 slice
Paste with grilled eggplant (Wawrzyniec)	58	40 g	2 tbsp

Kcal: 193 • P: 5 g • F: 8 g • C: 30 g • P: 77 mg • K: 216 mg • Na: 354 mg

Sandwich with eggplant paste

Preparation:

1. Spread the sandwich with vegetable paste.

DAY 8

Energy: 1588 kcal • Protein: 46 g • Fat: 55 g • Carbohydrates: 238 g • Phosphorus: 918.43 mg • Potassium: 2426.3 mg • Sodium: 2714.04 mg

Diet: 5 meals | 2000 kcal | B: 50 g | low protein

Breakfast

Product	Kcal	Weight	Home measure	
Rice milk	94	200 g	200 ml	
Semolina	173	48 g	4 tbsp	
Coconut shreds	119	18 g	3 tbsp	
Raspberries	62	120 g		2 handful
Maple syrup	14	5 g	1tsp	

Kcal: 462 • P: 9 g • F: 15 g • C: 75 g • P: 249 mg • K: 433 mg • Na: 87 mg

Coconut semolina with fruit

Preparation:

1. Boil milk and add semolina and 2 tablespoons of coconut shavings stir all the time.

2. Transfer to a bowl, add fruit and top with maple syrup. Sprinkle with the remaining roasted coconut shavings.

Second breakfast

Product	Kcal	Weight	Home measure
Wheat roll	218	80 g	1 piece
Butter	50	7 g	1tsp
Ricotta cheese	30	20 g	1 tbsp
Strawberry jam low-sugar	15	10 g	1tsp

Kcal: 314 • P: 8 g • F: 9 g • C: 51 g • P: 92 mg • K: 141 mg • Na: 326 mg

Wheat bun with cottage cheese and jam

Preparation:

1. Cut roll in half, spread with butter, cheese and jam.

Lunch

Product	Kcal	Weight	Home measure
Chickpea flour (besan)	232	60 g	5 tbsp
Water	0	70 g	70ml
Olive oil	44	5 g	1tsp
Baking soda	0	2 g	0.5 tsp
Salt	0	1 g	1 pinch
Pepper black	3	1 g	1 pinch
Avocado	48	30 g	2 slice
Red onion	8	20 g	1 slice
Lime juice	2	6 g	2tsp
Pepper red	10	40 g	small 0.5 piece
Carrot	12	36 g	large 0.5 piece
Cucumber	8	50 g	10 slice
Red beans canned	16	20 g	1 tbsp
Radish sprouts	2	4 g	0.5 tbsp

Kcal: 385 • P: 17 g • F: 14 g • C: 51 g • P: 322 mg • K: 1031 mg • Na: 1057 mg

Vegan tortilla with vegetables

Preparation:

1. Mix ingredients for tortilla (flour, water, oil, soda, salt, pepper) thoroughly.

2. Heat a pancake pan. Add dough and fry until it is thickened, flip to other side and fry for a while more.
3. Mash avocado. Add spices, chopped red onion, lime juice and mix everything thoroughly.
4. Spread tortilla with avocado paste, add vegetables cut into bars, drained beans, sprouts and wrap.

Snack

Product	Kcal	Weight	Home measure
Carrot	46	140 g	large 2 piece
Pear	107	160 g	small 1 piece
Lemon juice	1	6 g	1 tbsp
Walnuts	98	15 g	1 tbsp

Kcal: 253 • P: 4 g • F: 10 g • C: 40 g • P: 124 mg • K: 716 mg • Na: 99 mg

Carrot salad and nuts

Preparation:

1. Wash, peel and grate carrots on a coarse grater.

2. Dice peeled pear, sprinkle with lemon juice, add carrots and mix.

3. Sprinkle the top with chopped nuts.

Dinner

Product	Kcal	Weight	Home measure
Rye bread	91	35 g	1 slice
Vegan slices with pistachios (Go Vege)	13	12 g	1 slice
Royal cheese	53	15 g	1 slice
Mustard	10	10 g	1tsp
Sprouts mix	5	8 g	1 tbsp
Pickled cucumber	4	37 g	small 1 piece

Kcal: 176 • P: 8 g • F: 7 g • C: 21 g • P: 131 mg • K: 105 mg • Na: 1146 mg

Toast with ham and cheese

Preparation:

1. Toast bread in a toaster or toaster oven.

2. Brush toast with mustard, put vegan "ham", cheese and vegetables.

DAY 9

Energy: 1982 kcal • Protein: 48 g • Fat: 73 g • Carbohydrates: 303 g • Phosphorus: 999.45 mg • Potassium: 2401.2 mg • Sodium: 1068.38 mg

Diet: 5 meals | 2000 kcal | B: 50 g | low protein

Breakfast

Product	Kcal	Weight	Home measure
Oat flakes	152	40 g	4 tbsp
Coconut yogurt	118	125 g	5 tbsp
Natural yogurt 2%	24	40 g	2 tbsp
Pineapple	108	240 g	3 slice
Coconut shreds	40	6 g	1 tbsp

Kcal: 441 • P: 10 g • F: 16 g • C: 68 g • P: 247 mg • K: 557 mg • Na: 42 mg

Oatmeal with pineapple

Preparation:

1. Pour flakes into a saucepan, water, cook about 5- 6 minutes stirring.

2. To finished oatmeal add remaining ingredients.

Second breakfast

Product	Kcal	Weight	Home measure
Light rye bread	75	30 g	1 slice
Mango	54	90 g	2 slice
Turkey ham	33	30 g	2 slice
Lettuce butterhead	8	60 g	2 handful
Lemon juice	5	24 g	4 tbsp
Olive oil	133	15 g	3tsp

Kcal: 308 • P: 11 g • F: 17 g • C: 34 g • P: 159 mg • K: 445 mg • Na: 458 mg

Turkey and mango salad

Preparation:

1. Toast bread in a toaster oven and cut and dice.

2. Dice mango and ham, and tear lettuce into smaller pieces.

3. Mix all ingredients.

4. Pour dressing prepared from lemon juice and olive oil over salad. Sprinkle croutons on top.

Lunch

Product	Kcal	Weight	Home measure
Corn pasta	214	60 g	60g
Onion	12	35 g	small 0.5 piece
Olive oil	133	15 g	3tsp
Spinach frozen	29	100 g	100g
Chickpeas in brine	127	100 g	5 tbsp
Basil pesto	74	20 g	1 tbsp
Garlic	6	4 g	1 clove

Kcal: 595 • P: 17 g • F: 27 g • C: 72 g • P: 316 mg • K: 764 mg • Na: 416 mg

Pasta with chickpea pesto

Preparation:

1. Cook pasta according to the recipe on the package.

3. Dice onion and fry in olive oil.

4. Add spinach and simmer for about 10 minutes.

5. Drain chickpeas and add them to pan.

5. Mix pasta with pesto and pressed garlic and simmer
for 5 min.

doktorbarbara.pl

Snack

Product	Kcal	Weight	Home measure
Apple	104	200 g	large
Honey	36	12 g	1 piece 1tsp
Walnuts	98	15 g	1 tbsp
Cinnamon ground	5	2 g	0.5 tsp

Kcal: 244 • P: 3 g • F: 10 g • C: 41 g • P: 76 mg • K: 295 mg • Na: 3 mg

Baked apple with cinnamon, nuts and honey

Preparation:

1. Bake apple in oven.

2. Add rest of ingredients.

Dinner

Product	Kcal	Weight	Home measure
Rice noodles	218	60 g	60g
Raspberries	62	120 g	2 handful
Natural yogurt 2%	37	60 g	3 tbsp
Honey	73	24 g	2tsp
Cinnamon ground	5	2 g	0.5 tsp

Kcal: 395 • P: 8 g • F: 2 g • C: 88 g • P: 202 mg • K: 340 mg • Na: 149 mg

Pasta with raspberry sauce

Preparation:

1. Cook pasta according to the instructions on the package.

2. Crush raspberries, add yogurt and honey, mix.

3. Pour sauce over pasta, sprinkle with cinnamon.

DAY 10

Energy: 2088 kcal • Protein: 47 g • Fat: 63 g • Carbohydrates: 349 g • Phosphorus: 868.06 mg • Potassium: 2690.32 mg • Sodium: 2333.91 mg

Diet:5 meals | 2000 kcal | B: 50 g | low protein

Breakfast

Product	Kcal	Weight	Home measure
Buttery croissant (Lidl)	322	100 g	1 piece
Butter	50	7 g	1tsp
Strawberry jam low-sugar	76	50 g	5tsp

Kcal: 448 • P: 9 g • F: 11 g • C: 77 g • P: 5 mg • K: 31 mg • Na: 1 mg

Buttery croissant with jam

Preparation:

1. Cut the roll in half. Spread with butter and jam.

e-mail: **bp@doktorbarbara.pl**   Page 19

Second breakfast

Product	Kcal	Weight	Home measure
Vegetable broth	50	500 g	2 glass
Broccoli	93	300 g	300g
Olive oil	177	20 g	2 tbsp
Almonds flakes	116	20 g	2 tbsp
Garlic	18	12 g	3 clove
Light rye bread	175	70 g	2.3 slice
Basil fresh	2	10 g	1 handful

Kcal: 631 • P: 18 g • F: 35 g • C: 74 g • P: 406 mg • K: 1591 mg • Na: 1950 mg

1 servings:
Kcal: 315 • P: 9 g • F: 17 g • C: 37 g • P: 203 mg • K: 795 mg • Na: 975 mg

Broccoli soup with toast 🌙

Multiple servings recipe - 1/2 servings

Preparation:

1. Add broccoli florets and pressed garlic to boiling vegetable stock.

2. Cook until broccoli is tender.

3. Season to taste,

4. Blend the soup into a cream with 2 tablespoons of olive oil. Sprinkle with roasted almond flakes.

5. Toast the bread in a toaster oven. Mix the remaining olive oil with basil. Spread the oil on the croutons.

Lunch

Product	Kcal	Weight	Home measure
Rice noodles	655	180 g	180g
Onion	23	70 g	small 1 piece
Canola oil	177	20 g	2 tbsp
Garlic	12	8 g	2 clove
Zucchini	42	200 g	medium 0.5 piece
Canned chopped tomatoes	96	300 g	300g
Chickpeas in brine	152	120 g	6 tbsp
Salt	0	1 g	1 pinch
Parsley leaves	9	24 g	2 tbsp

Kcal: 1166 • P: 32 g • F: 26 g • C: 199 g • P: 700 mg • K: 2274 mg • Na: 1455 mg

1 servings:
Kcal: 583 • P: 16 g • F: 13 g • C: 100 g • P: 350 mg • K: 1137 mg • Na: 728 mg

Vegan cureo with pasta 🌙

Multiple servings recipe - 1/2 servings

Preparation:

1. Cook pasta according to the instructions on the package.

2. Peel, chop and fry onion in oil along with the garlic in a large pot.

3. Cut zucchini into cubes.

4. Add canned tomatoes, chickpeas to pan and simmer for 15 minutes.

5. Add some water, if necessary.

6. Finally, add salt, season and sprinkle with parsley .

Snack

Product	Kcal	Weight	Home measure
Hummus	142	60 g	3 tbsp
Light rye bread	150	60 g	2 slice
Radish sprouts	10	24 g	3 tbsp

Kcal: 303 • P: 8 g • F: 12 g • C: 44 g • P: 211 mg • K: 307 mg • Na: 619 mg

Sandwiches with hummus

Preparation:

1. Spread paste on the bread.

2. Decorate sandwiches with sprouts.

Dinner

Product	Kcal	Weight	Home measure
White rice	210	60 g	4 tbsp
Apple	146	280 g	2 piece medium
Cinnamon ground	5	2 g	0.5 tsp
Coconut shreds	79	12 g	2 tbsp

Kcal: 440 • P: 6 g • F: 9 g • C: 90 g • P: 99 mg • K: 420 mg • Na: 12 mg

Rice with apple and coconut chips

Preparation:

1. Cook rice according to the instructions on the package. 2. Grate apple and combine whole thing, adding cinnamon.

3. Sprinkle whole thing with coconut shavings.

DAY 11

Energy: 1657 kcal • Protein: 49 g • Fat: 58 g • Carbohydrates: 255 g • Phosphorus: 1366.37 mg • Potassium: 3827.48 mg • Sodium: 2119.08 mg

Diet:5 meals | 2000 kcal | B: 50 g | low protein

Breakfast

Product	Kcal	Weight	Home measure
Rice milk	94	200 g	200 ml
Semolina	173	48 g	4 tbsp
Coconut shreds	119	18 g	3 tbsp
Raspberries	62	120 g	2 handful
Maple syrup	14	5 g	1tsp

Kcal: 462 • P: 9 g • F: 15 g • C: 75 g • P: 249 mg • K: 433 mg • Na: 87 mg

Coconut semolina with fruit

Preparation:

1. Boil milk and add semolina and 2 tablespoons of coconut shavings stir all the time.

2. Transfer to a bowl, add fruit and top with maple syrup. Sprinkle with the remaining roasted coconut shavings.

Second breakfast

Product	Kcal	Weight	Home measure
Light rye bread	150	60 g	2 slice
Butter	50	7 g	1tsp
Italian style cheese Capri (Sierpc)	38	20 g	2tsp
Red tomato	22	120 g	1 piece medium
Onions green spring or scallions	5	15 g	1 piece medium
Olive oil	44	5 g	1tsp
Salt	0	1 g	1 pinch
Pepper black	3	1 g	1 pinch

Kcal: 311 • P: 6 g • F: 15 g • C: 42 g • P: 113 mg • K: 441 mg • Na: 799 mg

Italian sandwiches

Preparation:

1. Spread butter on sandwiches, add sliced Capri cheese.

2. Cut tomato into eights, mix with sliced onion. Drizzle the whole thing with olive oil, season.

Lunch

Product	Kcal	Weight	Home measure
Pumpkin	62	240 g	2 slice
Carrot	40	120 g	medium 2 piece
Onion	23	70 g	small 1 piece
Olive oil	44	5 g	1tsp
Chard	34	135 g	0.5 serving
Vanilla beans	6	2 g	0.5 tsp
Salt	0	2 g	2 pinch
Pepper black	5	2 g	1tsp
Pumpkin seeds	57	10 g	1 tbsp

Kcal: 270 • P: 10 g • F: 11 g • C: 43 g • P: 359 mg • K: 1848 mg • Na: 932 mg

Cream of pumpkin

Preparation:

1. Peel and dice pumpkin and carrot.

2. Fry onion in olive oil.

3. Add pumpkin and carrots.

4. Fry for about 10 minutes.

5. Cook vegetable stock.

6. Pour broth over pumpkin and carrots.

7. Cook until vegetables are soft.

8. Add vanilla bean.

9. Blend to smooth cream.

10. Season with salt and pepper, garnish with pumpkin seeds.

Snack

Product	Kcal	Weight	Home measure
Oat flakes	61	16 g	4tsp
Kiwi	46	75 g	1 piece
Strawberries	45	140 g	2 handful
Rice milk	94	200 g	200 ml
Cinnamon ground	10	4 g	1tsp

Kcal: 255 • P: 5 g • F: 4 g • C: 54 g • P: 239 mg • K: 577 mg • Na: 83 mg

Oat and rice smoothie

Preparation:

1. Pour boiling water over oatmeal, set aside for 3 minutes and blend with rest of ingredients.

2. If necessary, add water.

Dinner

Product	Kcal	Weight	Home measure
Egg	140	100 g	medium 2 piece
Milk 2%	23	45 g	3 tbsp
Oat flour	121	30 g	3 tbsp
Vanilla pudding without sugar	30	8 g	2tsp
Strawberries	45	140 g	2 handful

Kcal: 359 • P: 19 g • F: 14 g • C: 41 g • P: 406 mg • K: 529 mg • Na: 218 mg

Pudding omelette

Preparation:

1. Break the eggs, separate the whites from the yolks. Beat egg whites with a pinch of salt until stiff. In a bowl, mix egg yolks with milk, flour and pudding powder. Then add the egg whites in batches, mixing gently each time.

2. Pour the egg and pudding mixture into a non-fat frying pan, spread it evenly, reduce the heat and cook for a few minutes.

3. Slide the bottom-fried omelette onto a large plate, cover it with the pan and flip it over so that the un-fried side is on the bottom of the pan.

4. Fry for about 2 minutes.

5. Serve the omelette with fruit.

DAY 12

Energy: 2019 kcal • Protein: 49 g • Fat: 60 g • Carbohydrates: 338 g • Phosphorus: 1257.78 mg • Potassium: 2623.97 mg • Sodium: 2151.93 mg

Diet: 5 meals | 2000 kcal | B: 50 g | low protein

Breakfast

Product	Kcal	Weight	Home measure
Oat flakes	190	50 g	5 tbsp
Pear	107	160 g	small 1 piece
Honey	36	12 g	1tsp
Cinnamon ground	5	2 g	2 pinch
Coconut yogurt	47	50 g	2 tbsp
Natural yogurt 2%	24	40 g	2 tbsp
Walnuts	52	8 g	2 piece

Kcal: 462 • P: 11 g • F: 13 g • C: 78 g • P: 306 mg • K: 506 mg • Na: 35 mg

Oatmeal with pear and walnuts

Preparation:

1. Boil cereal in water.

2. Dice the pear, put it in a separate pot, add cinnamon and honey.

3. Pour a small amount of water to cover the fruit.

4. Cook for about 10 minutes, until the pear is soft.

5. Transfer oatmeal to a plate, top with the cooked fruit, yogurt, and nuts.

Second breakfast

Product	Kcal	Weight	Home measure
Natural yogurt	92	150 g	small 1 packaging
2% Corn flakes	214	60 g	2 serving

Kcal: 306 • P: 11 g • F: 3 g • C: 60 g • P: 244 mg • K: 401 mg • Na: 532 mg

Yogurt with corn flakes

Preparation:

1. Mix yogurt with flakes.

Lunch

Product	Kcal	Weight	Home measure
Corn pasta	357	100 g	100g
Tomatoes cherry	11	60 g	3 piece
Basil pesto	149	40 g	2 tbsp
Arugula	4	20 g	1 handful
Parmesan cheese	63	16 g	2 tbsp

Kcal: 583 • P: 16 g • F: 21 g • C: 86 g • P: 429 mg • K: 603 mg • Na: 611 mg

Pasta with pesto and tomatoes

Preparation:

1. Cook pasta according to the instructions on the package.

2. Cut tomatoes in half.

3. Mix pesto with warm pasta and tomatoes.

4. Sprinkle with grated cheese and add arugula.

Snack

Product	Kcal	Weight	Home measure
Strawberries	22	70 g	1 handful
Raspberries	31	60 g	1 handful
Blueberries	29	50 g	1 handful
Gelatin desserts dry mix	164	43 g	0.5 packaging
Natural yogurt 2%	12	20 g	1 tbsp

Kcal: 258 • P: 6 g • F: 1 g • C: 60 g • P: 125 mg • K: 279 mg • Na: 215 mg

Fruit in jelly

Preparation:

1. Prepare jelly according to the instructions on package.

2. Wash the fruits and pour over jelly. Put in refrigerator to let jelly set.

3. Add yogurt on top of dessert.

Dinner

Product	Kcal	Weight	Home measure
Avocado	112	70 g	0.5 piece
Lemon juice	1	6 g	1 tbsp
Olive oil	88	10 g	1 tbsp
Salt	0	1 g	1 pinch
Pepper black	3	1 g	1 pinch
Light rye bread	150	60 g	2 slice
Red tomato	11	60 g	medium 0.5 piece
Kiwi	46	75 g	1 piece

Kcal: 411 • P: 5 g • F: 22 g • C: 55 g • P: 153 mg • K: 835 mg • Na: 760 mg

Toast with avocado, kiwi

Preparation:

1. Mash avocado with a fork. Add lemon juice, olive oil, salt and pepper, mix.

2. Spread the bread slices with paste, add tomato slices.

3. Eat fruit separately.

DAY 13

Energy: 1972 kcal • Protein: 52 g • Fat: 83 g • Carbohydrates: 269 g • Phosphorus: 848.14 mg • Potassium: 2912.19 mg • Sodium: 806.39 mg

Diet:5 meals | 2000 kcal | B: 50 g | low protein

Breakfast

Product	Kcal	Weight	Home measure
White rice	210	60 g	4 tbsp
Pear	107	160 g	small 1 piece
Ginger ground	7	2 g	1tsp
Cinnamon ground	2	1 g	1 pinch
Turmeric ground	3	1 g	1 pinch
Coconut shreds	119	18 g	3 tbsp

Kcal: 448 • P: 6 g • F: 12 g • C: 80 g • P: 109 mg • K: 391 mg • Na: 13 mg

Spiced rice with pear

Preparation:

1. Cook rice according to the instructions on the package. 2. Cut fruit into cubes. Mix with spices.

3. Put rice on a plate add pear and coconut shavings.

Second breakfast

Product	Kcal	Weight	Home measure
Coconut yogurt	150	160 g	1 packaging
Raspberries	31	60 g	1 handful
Coconut shreds	79	12 g	2 tbsp
Walnuts	52	8 g	2 piece

Kcal: 313 • P: 4 g • F: 25 g • C: 22 g • P: 70 mg • K: 191 mg • Na: 18 mg

Coconut yogurt with raspberries

Preparation:

1. Mix yogurt with all ingredients.

Lunch

Product	Kcal	Weight	Home measure
Chicken breast	96	80 g	80g
Olive oil	177	20 g	2 tbsp
Pepper black	3	1 g	1 pinch
Turmeric ground	3	1 g	1 pinch
Leek	18	30 g	30g
Carrot	17	50 g	small 1 piece
Parsley root	14	40 g	0.5 piece
Celery root	18	60 g	1 slice
Potatoes	116	200 g	small 4 piece
Butter	100	14 g	2tsp

Kcal: 562 • P: 26 g • F: 34 g • C: 42 g • P: 375 mg • K: 1746 mg • Na: 181 mg

Chicken with vegetables and potatoes

Preparation:

1. Brush chicken with olive oil and rub with spices.

2. Cut leek into rings, peel and grate remaining vegetables (except the potatoes) on a coarse grater.

3. Steam chicken and vegetables for about 20 minutes or bake in foil.

4. Boil potatoes in water.

5. Serve chicken with vegetables and potatoes topped with butter.

Snack

Product	Kcal	Weight	Home measure
Light rye bread	150	60 g	2 slice
Italian style cheese Capri (Sierpc)	75	40 g	4tsp
Avocado	24	15 g	1 slice
Lettuce butterhead	4	30 g	1 handful

Kcal: 253 • P: 8 g • F: 9 g • C: 38 g • P: 93 mg • K: 244 mg • Na: 444 mg

Capri cheese and lettuce sandwiches

Preparation:

1. Spread the sandwiches with capri cheese.

2. Add lettuce and sliced avocado.

Dinner

Product	Kcal	Weight	Home measure
Rice noodles	218	60 g	60g
Raspberries	62	120 g	2 handful
Natural yogurt 2%	37	60 g	3 tbsp
Honey	73	24 g	2tsp
Cinnamon ground	5	2 g	0.5 tsp

Kcal: 395 • P: 8 g • F: 2 g • C: 88 g • P: 202 mg • K: 340 mg • Na: 149 mg

Pasta with raspberry sauce

Preparation:

1. Cook pasta according to the instructions on the package.

2. Crush raspberries, add yogurt and honey, mix.

3. Pour sauce over pasta, sprinkle with cinnamon.

DAY 14

Energy: 1815 kcal • Protein: 52 g • Fat: 56 g • Carbohydrates: 299 g • Phosphorus: 1156 mg • Potassium: 2940.49 mg • Sodium: 1441.67 mg

Diet:5 meals | 2000 kcal | B: 50 g | low protein

Breakfast

Product	Kcal	Weight	Home measure
Oat flakes	190	50 g	5 tbsp
Pear	107	160 g	small 1 piece
Honey	36	12 g	1tsp
Cinnamon ground	5	2 g	2 pinch
Coconut yogurt	47	50 g	2 tbsp
Natural yogurt 2%	24	40 g	2 tbsp
Walnuts	52	8 g	2 piece

Kcal: 462 • P: 11 g • F: 13 g • C: 78 g • P: 306 mg • K: 506 mg • Na: 35 mg

Oatmeal with pear and walnuts

Preparation:

1. Boil cereal in water.

2. Dice the pear, put it in a separate pot, add cinnamon and honey.

3. Pour a small amount of water to cover the fruit.

4. Cook for about 10 minutes, until the pear is soft.

5. Transfer oatmeal to a plate, top with the cooked fruit, yogurt, and nuts.

Second breakfast

Product	Kcal	Weight	Home measure
Light rye bread	75	30 g	1 slice
Mango	54	90 g	2 slice
Turkey ham	33	30 g	2 slice
Lettuce butterhead	8	60 g	2 handful
Lemon juice	5	24 g	4 tbsp
Olive oil	133	15 g	3tsp

Kcal: 308 • P: 11 g • F: 17 g • C: 34 g • P: 159 mg • K: 445 mg • Na: 458 mg

Turkey and mango salad

Preparation:

1. Toast bread in a toaster oven and cut and dice.

2. Dice mango and ham, and tear lettuce into smaller pieces.

3. Mix all ingredients.

4. Pour dressing prepared from lemon juice and olive oil over salad. Sprinkle croutons on top.

Lunch

Product	Kcal	Weight	Home measure
Millet	227	60 g	4 tbsp
Zucchini	17	80 g	8 slice
Button mushrooms	7	30 g	small 3 piece
Carrot	17	50 g	small 1 piece
Vegetable broth	13	125 g	0.5 glass
Egg	70	50 g	medium 1 piece
Parsley leaves	4	12 g	1 tbsp
Salt	0	1 g	1 pinch
Pepper black	3	1 g	1 pinch
Herbes de provence spice	3	1 g	1 pinch
Lettuce butterhead	4	30 g	1 handful
Natural yogurt 2%	12	20 g	1 tbsp

Kcal: 375 • P: 18 g • F: 9 g • C: 58 g • P: 431 mg • K: 1024 mg • Na: 891 mg

Baked vegetable cutlets

Preparation:

1. Rinse groats with boiling water, then cook according to the instructions on the package.

2. Grate zucchini and drain excess water.

3. Chop mushrooms, grate carrot and simmer vegetables
with addition of stock.

4. Add vegetables and egg to the cooled groats. Mix and season with chopped parsley, salt, pepper and herbs.
5. Form cutlets. Place them on a baking sheet lined with baking paper and bake for about 25 minutes at 200 degrees.

6. Serve cutlets on lettuce with yogurt.

Snack

Product	Kcal	Weight	Home measure
Coconut yogurt	75	80 g	0.5 packaging
Natural yogurt 2%	37	60 g	3 tbsp
Cocoa powder	11	5 g	1tsp
Blueberries	29	50 g	1 handful
Nectarine	48	110 g	small 1 piece
Raspberries	31	60 g	1 handful

Kcal: 231 • P: 7 g • F: 8 g • C: 38 g • P: 162 mg • K: 546 mg • Na: 46 mg

Yogurt with fruit

Preparation:

1. Mix yogurt with remaining ingredients.

Dinner

Product	Kcal	Weight	Home measure
White rice	210	60 g	4 tbsp
Apple	146	280 g	medium 2 piece
Cinnamon ground	5	2 g	0.5 tsp
Coconut shreds	79	12 g	2 tbsp

Kcal: 440 • P: 6 g • F: 9 g • C: 90 g • P: 99 mg • K: 420 mg • Na: 12 mg

Rice with apple and coconut chips

Preparation:

1. Cook rice according to the instructions on the package. 2. Grate apple and combine whole thing, adding cinnamon.
3. Sprinkle whole thing with coconut shavings.

SHOPPING LIST

Grocery list 1   25.01-31.01.2024

Baked products

Biscuits	63 g	21 small piece

Beans

Chickpeas canned	120 g	6 tbsp
Chickpeas in brine	120 g	6 tbsp
Green beans frozen	50 g	1 handful

Beverages

Lemon juice	90 g	15 tbsp
Lime juice	9 g	3 tsp
Water	615 g	2.5 glass

Brand foods

Coconut milk canned 19%	50 g	5 tbsp
Coconut milk canned light 6%	120 g	0.5 glass

Bread

Buttery croissant)	100 g	1 piece
Light rye bread	610 g	20.3 slice
Wheat roll	80 g	1 piece
Wheat-rye bread	60 g	2 slice

Breakfast cereals

Oat flakes	40 g	4 tbsp

Cereal products

Corn pasta	250 g	3.1 glass

Corn sweet canned	30 g	30 g
Jasmine rice	50 g	5 tbsp
Millet	75 g	5 tbsp
Rice flour white	100 g	10 tbsp
Rice noodles	240 g	4.8 serving
Semolina	48 g	4tbsp
Wheat white flour	120 g	8 tbsp
White rice	110 g	

Dairy

Italian style cheese Capri (Sierpc)	90 g	9 tsp
Mozzarella cheese	30 g	2 slice
Natural yogurt 2%	220 g	11 tbsp
Parmesan cheese	32 g	8 tsp
Quark half-fat	60 g	2 slice
Ricotta cheese	180 g	9 tbsp

Eggs

Egg	50 g	1 medium piece

Fats and oils

Butter	63g	9 tsp
Canola oil	80g	8 tbsp
Olive oil	95g	9.5 tbsp

Fish

Atlantic salmon80 g 0.4 piece

Foods for vegetarians and vegans

Coconut yogurt525 g 21 tbsp

Rice milk200 g 0.8 glass

Fruits

Apple280 g 2.5 small piece

Avocado225 g 15 slice

Banana100 g 1 small piece

Blueberries150 g 3 handful

Kiwi75 g 1 piece

Mango90 g 2 slice

Nectarine110 g 1 small piece

Orange240 g 1.5 small piece

Pear160 g 1 small piece

Pineapple350 g 4.4 slice

Raisins seedless9 g 0.3 handful

Raspberries540 g 9 handful

Strawberries70 g 1 handful

Meat

Turkey ham45 g

3 slice

Nuts and seeds

Almonds	10 g	10 piece
Almonds flakes	20 g	2 tbsp
Coconut shreds	66 g	11 tbsp
Linseed	5 g	1 tsp
Sesame	5 g	0.5 tbsp
Walnuts	16 g	0.5 handful

Sauces

Basil pesto	80 g	4 tbsp

Soups

Broth	150 g	0.6 glass
Vegetable broth	500 g	2 glass

Spices and herbs

Allspice spice	1 g	1 grain
Basil fresh	20 g	2 handful
Bay leaf	1 g	1 leaf
Cinnamon ground	3 g	3 pinch
Cocoa powder	5 g	0.5 tbsp
Coriander leaves	5 g	0.5handful
Dill fresh	25 g	5 tsp
Garlic	25 g	6.3 clove
Ginger ground	2 g	1 tsp
Ginger root	8 g	4 tsp
Horseraddish grated	4 g	1 tsp
Parsley leaves	60 g	5 tbsp
Pepper black	9 g	9 pinch
Salt	8 g	8 pinch
Sweet pepper spice	1 g	0.3 tsp
Turmeric ground	3 g	3 pinch

Spreads and pastes

Coconut cream	10 g	0.5 tbsp
Curry paste	5 g	0.3 tbsp
Hummus	120 g	6 tbsp
Paste with grilled eggplant (Wawrzyniec)	40 g	2 tbsp
Strawberry jam low-sugar	60 g	6 tsp

Sweets

Gelatin desserts dry mix	43 g	4.8 tsp

Honey	24 g	2 tsp
Maple syrup	15 g	3 tsp

Vegetables

Arugula	60 g	3 handful
Beets cooked	240 g	2 piece
Broccoli	350 g	17.5 floret
Button mushrooms	50 g	5 small piece
Cabbage chinese pe-tsai	100 g	2 leaf
Canned chopped tomatoes	300 g	0.8 can
Carrot	130 g	2.2medium piece
Cauliflower	105 g	7 floret
Celery	23 g	0.5 piece
Leek	50 g	1 piece
Lettuce butterhead	160 g	5.3 handful
Onion	175 g	2.5 small piece
Onions green spring or scallions	15 g	2.5 tbsp
Parsley root	40 g	0.5 piece
Pepper red	98 g	1.3 small piece
Peppers hot red chili	5 g	0.1 piece
Pickled cucumber	130 g	2 medium piece
Potatoes	420 g	8.4 small piece
Radish	30 g	2 piece
Radish sprouts	48 g	6 tbsp
Red tomato	410 g	2.4 piece
Shallot	20 g	2 tbsp

Spinach	100 g	4 handful	Zucchini	280 g	28 slice
Tomatoes cherry	120 g	1.2 handful			

Grocery list 2   01.02-07.02.2024

Baked products

Baking soda	2 g	0.5 tsp

Beans

Chickpeas in brine	220 g	11 tbsp
Red beans canned	20 g	1 tbsp

Beverages

Lemon juice	60 g	10 tbsp
Lime juice	6 g	2 tsp
Water	70 g	0.3 glass

Bread

Buttery croissant (Lidl)	100 g	1 piece
Light rye bread	370 g	12.3 slice
Rye bread	35 g	1 slice
Wheat roll	80 g	1 piece

Breakfast cereals

Corn flakes	60 g	20 tbsp
Oat flakes	156 g	15.6 tbsp

Cereal products

Chickpea flour (besan)	60 g	5 tbsp
Corn pasta	160 g	2glass
Millet	60 g	4 tbsp
Oat flour	30 g	3 tbsp

Rice noodles	300	6 serving
Semolina	96 g	8 tbsp
White rice	180g	180 g

Dairy

Italian style cheese Capri (Sierpc)	60 g	6 tsp
Milk 2%	45 g	0.2 glass
Natural yogurt 2%	490 g	24.5 tbsp
Parmesan cheese	16 g	4 tsp
Ricotta cheese	20 g	1 tbsp
Royal cheese	15 g	1 slice

Eggs

Egg	150 g	3 medium piece

Fats and oils

Butter	35 g	5 tsp
Canola oil	20 g	2 tbsp
Olive oil	110 g	11 tbsp

Foods for vegetarians and vegans

Coconut yogurt	465 g	18.6 tbsp
Rice milk	600 g	2.5 glass
Vegan slices with pistachios (Go Vege)	12 g	12 g

Fruits

Apple	760 g	6.9 small piece
Avocado	115 g	7.7 slice
Blueberries	100 g	2 handful
Kiwi	150 g	2 piece
Mango	180 g	4 slice
Nectarine	110 g	1 small piece
Pear	640 g	4 small piece
Pineapple	240 g	3 slice
Raspberries	660 g	11 handful
Strawberries	350 g	5 handful

Meat

Chicken breast	80 g	0.4 piece
Turkey ham	60 g	4 slice

Nuts and seeds

Almonds flakes	20 g	2 tbsp
Coconut shreds	96 g	16 tbsp
Pumpkin seeds	10 g	1 tbsp
Walnuts	54 g	1.8 handful

Sauces

Basil pesto	60 g	3 tbsp
Mustard	10 g	0.5 tbsp

Soups

Vegetable broth	625 g	2.5 glass

Spices and herbs

Basil fresh	10 g	1 handful
Cinnamon ground	19 g	19 pinch
Cocoa powder	5 g	0.5 tbsp
Garlic	24 g	6 clove
Ginger ground	2 g	1 tsp
Herbes de provence spice	1 g	0.3 tsp
Parsley leaves	36 g	3 tbsp
Pepper black	7 g	7 pinch
Salt	7 g	7 pinch
Turmeric ground	2 g	2 pinch
Vanilla beans	2 g	2 g

Spreads and pastes

Hummus	60 g	3 tbsp
Strawberry jam low-sugar	60 g	6 tsp

Sweets

Gelatin desserts dry mix	43 g	4.8 tsp
Honey	84 g	7 tsp
Maple syrup	10 g	2 tsp
Vanilla pudding without sugar	8 g	2 tsp

Vegetables

Arugula	20 g	1 handful
Broccoli	300 g	15 floret
Button mushrooms	30 g	3 small piece

Canned chopped tomatoes	300 g	0.8 can
Carrot	396 g	6.6 medium
Celery root	60 g	piece 1 slice
Chard	135 g	0.5 serving
Cucumber	50 g	0.3 piece
Leek	30 g	0.6 piece
Lettuce butterhead	180 g	6 handful
Onion	175 g	2.5 small piece
Onions green spring or scallions	15 g	2.5 tbsp
Parsley root	40 g	0.5 piece
Pepper red	40 g	0.5 small piece

Pickled cucumber	37 g	0.6 medium piece
Potatoes	200 g	4 small piece
Pumpkin	240 g	2 slice
Radish sprouts	28 g	3.5 tbsp
Red onion	20 g	0.2 piece
Red tomato	180 g	1.1 piece
Spinach frozen	100 g	2 serving
Sprouts mix	8 g	1 tbsp
Tomatoes cherry	60 g	0.6 handful
Zucchini	280 g	28 slice

MEAL LISTS

Diet: 5 meals | 2000 kcal | B: 50 g | low protein

BREAKFAST

Proposition 1

Product	Kcal	Weight	Home measure
Oat flakes	152	40 g	4 tbsp
Coconut yogurt	118	125 g	5 tbsp
Natural yogurt 2%	24	40 g	2 tbsp
Pineapple	108	240 g	3 slice
Coconut shreds	40	6 g	1 tbsp

Kcal: 441 • P: 10 g • F: 16 g • C: 68 g • P: 247 mg • K: 557 mg • Na: 42 mg

Oatmeal with pineapple

Preparation:

1. Pour flakes into a saucepan, water, cook about 5- 6 minutes stirring.

2. To finished oatmeal add remaining ingredients.

Proposition 2

Product	Kcal	Weight	Home measure
Lettuce butterhead	1	10 g	2 leaf
Apple	36	70 g	0.5 medium piece
Leek	31	50 g	1 piece
Dill fresh	2	5 g	1tsp
Orange	50	80 g	small
Olive oil	44	5 g	0.5 piece
Light rye bread	150	60 g	1tsp
Butter	100	14 g	2 slice
Italian style cheese Capri (Sierpc)	56	30 g	2tsp 3tsp

Kcal: 472 • P: 8 g • F: 22 g • C: 65 g • P: 128 mg • K: 485 mg • Na: 439 mg

Sandwiches and apple salad

Preparation:

1. wash and chop the lettuce.

2. Grate apple on a coarse grater.

3. Chop leek and dill finely.

4. Mix the vegetables with the apple. Add orange juice and oil.

5. Season to taste and set aside in the refrigerator for 30 minutes.

6. Prepare croutons from bread in a toaster oven or oven. Then spread with butter and add capri cheese.

7. Eat salad with croutons.

Proposition 3

Product	Kcal	Weight	Home measure
Cabbage chinese pe-tsai	16	100 g	100g
Red tomato	11	60 g	medium 0.5 piece
Onion	12	35 g	small 0.5 piece
Pepper red	10	38 g	small 0.5 piece
Corn sweet canned	19	30 g	2 tbsp
Olive oil	88	10 g	1 tbsp
Lemon juice	1	6 g	1 tbsp
Sweet pepper spice	3	1 g	1 pinch
Salt	0	1 g	1 pinch
Pepper black	3	1 g	1 pinch
Light rye bread	150	60 g	2 slice
Butter	100	14 g	2tsp
Turkey ham	17	15 g	1 slice

Kcal: 429 • P: 10 g • F: 24 g • C: 50 g • P: 205 mg • K: 721 mg • Na: 952 mg

Sandwiches and salad of Chinese cabbage

Preparation:

1. Chop vegetables and mix with olive oil, lemon juice and spices.

2. Spread bread with butter, add ham.

3. Sandwich eat with salad.

Proposition 4

Product	Kcal	Weight	Home measure
White rice	210	60 g	4 tbsp
Pear	107	160 g	small 1 piece
Ginger ground	7	2 g	1tsp
Cinnamon ground	2	1 g	1 pinch
Turmeric ground	3	1 g	1 pinch
Coconut shreds	119	18 g	3 tbsp

Kcal: 448 • P: 6 g • F: 12 g • C: 80 g • P: 109 mg • K: 391 mg • Na: 13 mg

Spiced rice with pear

Preparation:

1. Cook rice according to the instructions on the package. 2. Cut fruit into cubes. Mix with spices.

3. Put rice on a plate add pear and coconut shavings.

Proposition 5

Product	Kcal	Weight	Home measure
Buttery croissant (Lidl)	322	100 g	1 piece
Butter	50	7 g	1tsp
Strawberry jam low-sugar	76	50 g	5tsp

Kcal: 448 • P: 9 g • F: 11 g • C: 77 g • P: 5 mg • K: 31 mg • Na: 1 mg

Buttery croissant with jam

Preparation:

1. Cut the roll in half. Spread with butter and jam.

Proposition 6

Product	Kcal	Weight	Home measure
Rice milk	94	200 g	200 ml
Semolina	173	48 g	4 tbsp
Coconut shreds	119	18 g	3 tbsp
Raspberries	62	120 g	2 handful
Maple syrup	14	5 g	1tsp

Kcal: 462 • P: 9 g • F: 15 g • C: 75 g • P: 249 mg • K: 433 mg • Na: 87 mg

Coconut semolina with fruit

Preparation:

1. Boil milk and add semolina and 2 tablespoons of coconut shavings stir all the time.

2. Transfer to a bowl, add fruit and top with maple syrup. Sprinkle with the remaining roasted coconut shavings.

Proposition 7

Product	Kcal	Weight	Home measure
Oat flakes	190	50 g	5 tbsp
Pear	107	160 g	small 1 piece
Honey	36	12 g	1tsp
Cinnamon ground	5	2 g	2 pinch
Coconut yogurt	47	50 g	2 tbsp
Natural yogurt 2%	24	40 g	2 tbsp
Walnuts	52	8 g	2 piece

Kcal: 462 • P: 11 g • F: 13 g • C: 78 g • P: 306 mg • K: 506 mg • Na: 35 mg

Oatmeal with pear and walnuts

Preparation:

1. Boil cereal in water.

2. Dice the pear, put it in a separate pot, add cinnamon and honey.

3. Pour a small amount of water to cover the fruit.

4. Cook for about 10 minutes, until the pear is soft.

5. Transfer oatmeal to a plate, top with the cooked fruit, yogurt, and nuts.

Proposition 8

Product	Kcal	Weight	Home measure
Millet	170	45 g	3 tbsp
Apple	73	140 g	medium 1 piece
Water	0	15 g	1 tbsp
Raisins seedless	27	9 g	1 tbsp
Almonds	58	10 g	10 piece
Lemon juice	1	6 g	2tsp
Maple syrup	27	10 g	1 tbsp

Kcal: 356 • P: 8 g • F: 7 g • C: 69 g • P: 201 mg • K: 406 mg • Na: 7 mg

Sweet millet groats with apple

Preparation:

1. Rinse millet in cold water and cook it according to the recipe on the package.

2. Peel and slice apple and stew in a pot with a tablespoon of water for about 10 minutes.

3. Add raisins, chopped almonds and drizzle with

lemon juice.

4. Add millet and mix with the honey.

SECOND BREAKFAST

Proposition 1

Product	Kcal	Weight	Home measure
Vegetable broth	50	500 g	2 glass
Broccoli	93	300 g	300g
Olive oil	177	20 g	2 tbsp
Almonds flakes	116	20 g	2 tbsp
Garlic	18	12 g	3 clove
Light rye bread	175	70 g	2.3 slice
Basil fresh	2	10 g	1 handful

Kcal: 631 • P: 18 g • F: 35 g • C: 74 g • P: 406 mg • K: 1591 mg • Na: 1950 mg

1 servings:
Kcal: 315 • P: 9 g • F: 17 g • C: 37 g • P: 203 mg • K: 795 mg • Na: 975 mg

Broccoli soup with toast 🍜

Multiple servings recipe - 1/2 servings

Preparation:

1. Add broccoli florets and pressed garlic to boiling vegetable stock.

2. Cook until broccoli is tender.

3. Season to taste,

4. Blend the soup into a cream with 2 tablespoons of olive oil. Sprinkle with roasted almond flakes.
5. Toast the bread in a toaster oven. Mix the remaining olive oil with basil. Spread the oil on the croutons.

Proposition 2

Product	Kcal	Weight	Home measure
Wheat roll	218	80 g	1 piece
Butter	50	7 g	1tsp
Ricotta cheese	30	20 g	1 tbsp
Strawberry jam low-sugar	15	10 g	1tsp

Kcal: 314 • P: 8 g • F: 9 g • C: 51 g • P: 92 mg • K: 141 mg • Na: 326 mg

Wheat bun with cottage cheese and jam

Preparation:

1. Cut roll in half, spread with butter, cheese and jam.

Proposition 3

Product	Kcal	Weight	Home measure
Coconut yogurt	150	160 g	1 packaging
Raspberries	31	60 g	1 handful
Coconut shreds	79	12 g	2 tbsp
Walnuts	52	8 g	2 piece

Kcal: 313 • P: 4 g • F: 25 g • C: 22 g • P: 70 mg • K: 191 mg • Na: 18 mg

Coconut yogurt with raspberries

Preparation:

1. Mix yogurt with all ingredients.

Proposition 4

Product	Kcal	Weight	Home measure
Ricotta cheese	150	100 g	5 tbsp
Natural yogurt 2%	24	40 g	2 tbsp
Raspberries	31	60 g	1 handful
Blueberries	29	50 g	1 handful
Biscuits	68	18 g	large 2 piece

Kcal: 302 • P: 12 g • F: 12 g • C: 37 g • P: 257 mg • K: 448 mg • Na: 163 mg

Ricotta cheese with raspberries

Preparation:

1. Mix cheese with yogurt and fruit.

2. Eat with biscotti.

Proposition 5

Product	Kcal	Weight	Home measure
Light rye bread	75	30 g	1 slice
Mango	54	90 g	2 slice
Turkey ham	33	30 g	2 slice
Lettuce butterhead	8	60 g	2 handful
Lemon juice	5	24 g	4 tbsp
Olive oil	133	15 g	3tsp

Kcal: 308 • P: 11 g • F: 17 g • C: 34 g • P: 159 mg • K: 445 mg • Na: 458 mg

Turkey and mango salad

Preparation:

1. Toast bread in a toaster oven and cut and dice.

2. Dice mango and ham, and tear lettuce into smaller pieces.

3. Mix all ingredients.

4. Pour dressing prepared from lemon juice and olive oil over salad. Sprinkle croutons on top.

Proposition 6

Product	Kcal	Weight	Home measure
Light rye bread	150	60 g	2 slice
Butter	50	7 g	1tsp
Italian style cheese Capri (Sierpc)	38	20 g	2tsp
Red tomato	22	120 g	medium 1 piece
Onions green spring or scallions	5	15 g	medium 1 piece
Olive oil	44	5 g	1tsp
Salt	0	1 g	1 pinch
Pepper black	3	1 g	1 pinch

Kcal: 311 • P: 6 g • F: 15 g • C: 42 g • P: 113 mg • K: 441 mg • Na: 799 mg

Italian sandwiches

Preparation:

1. Spread butter on sandwiches, add sliced Capri cheese.

2. Cut tomato into eights, mix with sliced onion. Drizzle the whole thing with olive oil, season.

Proposition 7

Product	Kcal	Weight	Home measure
Natural yogurt	92	150 g	small
2% Corn flakes	214	60 g	1 packaging 2 serving

Kcal: 306 • P: 11 g • F: 3 g • C: 60 g • P: 244 mg • K: 401 mg • Na: 532 mg

Yogurt with corn flakes

Preparation:

1. Mix yogurt with flakes.

LUNCH

Proposition 1

Product	Kcal	Weight	Home measure
Chicken breast	96	80 g	80g
Olive oil	177	20 g	2 tbsp
Pepper black	3	1 g	1 pinch
Turmeric ground	3	1 g	1 pinch
Leek	18	30 g	30g
Carrot	17	50 g	small 1 piece
Parsley root	14	40 g	0.5 piece
Celery root	18	60 g	1 slice
Potatoes	116	200 g	small 4. piece
Butter	100	14 g	2tsp

Kcal: 562 • P: 26 g • F: 34 g • C: 42 g • P: 375 mg • K: 1746 mg • Na: 181 mg

Chicken with vegetables and potatoes

Preparation:

1. Brush chicken with olive oil and rub with spices.

2. Cut leek into rings, peel and grate remaining vegetables (except the potatoes) on a coarse grater.

3. Steam chicken and vegetables for about 20 minutes or bake in foil.

4. Boil potatoes in water.

5. Serve chicken with vegetables and potatoes topped with butter.

Proposition 2

Product	Kcal	Weight	Home measure
Atlantic salmon	166	80 g	80g
Lemon juice	1	6 g	1 tbsp
Sesame	29	5 g	1tsp
Potatoes	157	270 g	large 3 piece
Olive oil	88	10 g	1 tbsp
Dill fresh	4	10 g	1 tbsp
Apple	36	70 g	medium 0.5 piece
Carrot	17	50 g	small
Horseraddish grated	4	4 g	1 piece
Canola oil	88	10 g	1tsp
Salt	0	1 g	1 tbsp
Pepper black	3	1 g	1 pinch
			1 pinch

Kcal: 594 • P: 25 g • F: 34 g • C: 50 g • P: 360 mg • K: 1767 mg • Na: 523 mg

Grilled salmon with potatoes

Preparation:

1. Drizzle the salmon with lemon juice, coat with sesame seeds and grill for 3-4 minutes.

2. Doil the potatoes, then drizzle with olive oil and sprinkle with chopped dill.

3. Grate the apple and carrot on a small-mesh grater, mix with the chan and oil. Season.

4. Serve salmon with potatoes and carrot salad.

Proposition 3

Product	Kcal	Weight	Home measure
Corn pasta	357	100 g	100g
Tomatoes cherry	11	60 g	3 piece
Basil pesto	149	40 g	2 tbsp
Arugula	4	20 g	1 handful
Parmesan cheese	63	16 g	2 tbsp

Kcal: 583 • P: 16 g • F: 21 g • C: 86 g • P: 429 mg • K: 603 mg • Na: 611 mg

Pasta with pesto and tomatoes

Preparation:

1. Cook pasta according to the instructions on the package.

2. Cut tomatoes in half.

3. Mix pesto with warm pasta and tomatoes.

4. Sprinkle with grated cheese and add arugula.

Proposition 4

Product	Kcal	Weight	Home measure
Rice noodles	655	180 g	180g
Onion	23	70 g	small 1 piece
Canola oil	177	20 g	2 tbsp
Garlic	12	8 g	2 clove
Zucchini	42	200 g	medium 0.5 piece
Canned chopped tomatoes	96	300 g	300g
Chickpeas in brine	152	120 g	6 tbsp
Salt	0	1 g	1 pinch
Parsley leaves	9	24 g	2 tbsp

Kcal: 1166 • P: 32 g • F: 26 g • C: 199 g • P: 700 mg • K: 2274 mg • Na: 1455 mg

1 servings:
Kcal: 583 • P: 16 g • F: 13 g • C: 100 g • P: 350 mg • K: 1137 mg • Na: 728 mg

Vegan cureo with pasta 🌙

Multiple servings recipe - 1/2 servings

Preparation:

1. Cook pasta according to the instructions on the package.

2. Peel, chop and fry onion in oil along with the garlic in a large pot.

3. Cut zucchini into cubes.

4. Add canned tomatoes, chickpeas to pan and simmer for 15 minutes.

5. Add some water, if necessary.

6. Finally, add salt, season and sprinkle with parsley .

Proposition 5

Product	Kcal	Weight	Home measure
Potatoes	87	150 g	medium 2 piece
Onion	23	70 g	small 1 piece
Canola oil	265	30 g	3 tbsp
Quark half-fat	79	60 g	3 tbsp
Salt	0	1 g	1 pinch
Pepper black	5	2 g	2 pinch
Turmeric ground	6	2 g	1tsp
Wheat white flour	437	120 g	8 tbsp
Rice flour white	366	100 g	10 tbsp
Water	0	150 g	150 ml

Kcal: 1269 • P: 35 g • F: 36 g • C: 200 g • P: 450 mg • K: 1045 mg • Na: 438 mg

1 servings:
Kcal: 634 • P: 17 g • F: 18 g • C: 100 g • P: 225 mg • K: 522 mg • Na: 219 mg

Homemade dumplings 🌙

Multiple servings recipe - 1/2 servings

Preparation:

1. Peel and cut potatoes into smaller pieces. Transfer to a pot of water and cook until tender, about 20-25 minutes.

2. At this time, cut onions into small cubes and fry them in oil until browned.

3. Put cottage cheese into a bowl and mash it with a fork. Add the fried onions and mix.

4. Drain the boiled potatoes and add to bowl. Mash with a pestle until the ingredients are thoroughly combined.

5. Add spices, mix and set aside.

6. In a separate bowl, add flour (230 g) oil and salt, and finally hot water. Mix with a spoon and then knead dough with your hands.

7. Form a ball and divide it into 4 parts.

8. Dust the dough with the remaining flour. Roll it out, cut out circles with a glass.

9. Put 2 teaspoons of stuffing each on the dough pieces and seal the dumplings.

10. Drop half of dumplings into a pot of boiling water. Cook about 2 minutes from the moment they float to surface of the water.

Proposition 6

Product	Kcal	Weight	Home measure
Corn pasta	214	60 g	60g
Onion	12	35 g	small 0.5 piece
Olive oil	133	15 g	3tsp
Spinach frozen	29	100 g	100g
Chickpeas in brine	127	100 g	5 tbsp
Basil pesto	74	20 g	1 tbsp
Garlic	6	4 g	1 clove

Kcal: 595 • P: 17 g • F: 27 g • C: 72 g • P: 316 mg • K: 764 mg • Na: 416 mg

Pasta with chickpea pesto

Preparation:

1. Cook pasta according to the recipe on the package.

3. Dice onion and fry in olive oil.

4. Add spinach and simmer for about 10 minutes.

5. Drain chickpeas and add them to pan.

5. Mix pasta with pesto and pressed garlic and simmer for 5 min.

Proposition 7

Product	Kcal	Weight	Home measure
Olive oil	44	5 g	1tsp
Shallot	14	20 g	2 tbsp
Garlic	7	5 g	1.3 clove
Peppers hot red chili	2	5 g	1 piece
Ginger root	2	2 g	1tsp
Button mushrooms	11	50 g	small 5 piece
Curry paste	5	5 g	0.5 tsp
Coriander leaves	1	5 g	5 g
Zucchini	17	80 g	8 slice
Coconut milk canned 19%	94	50 g	5 tbsp
Water	0	200 g	200 ml
Broccoli	16	50 g	50g
Green beans frozen	17	50 g	1 handful
Chickpeas canned	106	120 g	6 tbsp
Spinach	4	25 g	1 handful
Lime juice	2	9 g	3tsp
Jasmine rice	174	50 g	5 tbsp

Kcal: 515 • P: 18 g • F: 18 g • C: 77 g • P: 305 mg • K: 1282 mg • Na: 339 mg

Vegetarian curry with chickpeas

Preparation:

1. Pour oil into large pot or wok, add sliced shallots, garlic, chili, ginger and simmer for about 3 minutes.

2. Add chopped vegetables, first mushrooms, after another 3 minutes add curry paste, a few sprigs of coriander and zucchini.

3. Simmer for about 4 minutes.

4. Pour in milk and 200 ml of water.

5. Cook for 5 minutes, add broccoli, beans and chickpeas.

6. After 5-6 minutes, add spinach and season with lime juice.

7. Serve with cooked rice and rest of coriander.

Proposition 8

Product	Kcal	Weight	Home measure
Millet	227	60 g	4 tbsp
Zucchini	17	80 g	8 slice
Button mushrooms	7	30 g	small 3 piece
Carrot	17	50 g	small 1 piece
Vegetable broth	13	125 g	0.5 glass
Egg	70	50 g	medium 1 piece
Parsley leaves	4	12 g	1 tbsp
Salt	0	1 g	1 pinch
Pepper black	3	1 g	1 pinch
Herbes de provence spice	3	1 g	1 pinch
Lettuce butterhead	4	30 g	1 handful
Natural yogurt 2%	12	20 g	1 tbsp

Kcal: 375 • P: 18 g • F: 9 g • C: 58 g • P: 431 mg • K: 1024 mg • Na: 891 mg

Baked vegetable cutlets

Preparation:

1. Rinse groats with boiling water, then cook according to the instructions on the package.

2. Grate zucchini and drain excess water.

3. Chop mushrooms, grate carrot and simmer vegetables
with addition of stock.

4. Add vegetables and egg to the cooled groats. Mix and season with chopped parsley, salt, pepper and herbs.

5. Form cutlets. Place them on a baking sheet lined with baking paper and bake for about 25 minutes at 200 degrees.

6. Serve cutlets on lettuce with yogurt.

Proposition 9

Product	Kcal	Weight	Home measure
Chickpea flour (besan)	232	60 g	5 tbsp
Water	0	70 g	70ml
Olive oil	44	5 g	1tsp
Baking soda	0	2 g	0.5 tsp
Salt	0	1 g	1 pinch
Pepper black	3	1 g	1 pinch
Avocado	48	30 g	2 slice
Red onion	8	20 g	1 slice
Lime juice	2	6 g	2tsp
Pepper red	10	40 g	small 0.5 piece
Carrot	12	36 g	large 0.5 piece
Cucumber	8	50 g	10 slice
Red beans canned	16	20 g	1 tbsp
Radish sprouts	2	4 g	0.5 tbsp

Kcal: 385 • P: 17 g • F: 14 g • C: 51 g • P: 322 mg • K: 1031 mg • Na: 1057 mg

Vegan tortilla with vegetables

Preparation:

1. Mix ingredients for tortilla (flour, water, oil, soda, salt, pepper) thoroughly.

2. Heat a pancake pan. Add dough and fry until it is thickened, flip to other side and fry for a while more.

3. Mash avocado. Add spices, chopped red onion, lime juice and mix everything thoroughly.

4. Spread tortilla with avocado paste, add vegetables cut into bars, drained beans, sprouts and wrap.

Proposition 10

Product	Kcal	Weight	Home measure
Carrot	10	30 g	medium 0,5 piece
Parsley root	14	40 g	0.5 piece
Celery	3	23 g	0.5 piece
Broth	74	150 g	150 ml
Pepper black	3	1 g	1 pinch
Salt	0	1 g	1 pinch
Dill fresh	4	10 g	2tsp
Millet	113	30 g	2 tbsp
Cauliflower	26	105 g	7 floret
Allspice spice	3	1 g	1 grain
Bay leaf	3	1 g	1 leaf
Olive oil	44	5 g	1tsp

Kcal: 297 • P: 16 g • F: 11 g • C: 37 g • P: 186 mg • K: 862 mg • Na: 1091 mg

Dill soup with cauliflower and millet

Preparation:

1. Peel, wash and dice carrots, parsley and celery.

2. Pour in broth, add water, bay leaves and allspice.

3. Boil under the lid for 15 minutes. Add cauliflower florets and cook for 5 minutes together.

4. Add millet and cook until tender.

5. Towards the end of cooking add olive oil and chopped dill.

6. Season soup to taste.

Proposition 11

Product	Kcal	Weight	Home measure
Pumpkin	62	240 g	2 slice
Carrot	40	120 g	medium 2. piece
Onion	23	70 g	small 1 piece
Olive oil	44	5 g	1tsp
Chard	34	135 g	0.5 serving
Vanilla beans	6	2 g	0.5 tsp
Salt	0	2 g	2 pinch
Pepper black	5	2 g	1tsp
Pumpkin seeds	57	10 g	1 tbsp

Kcal: 270 • P: 10 g • F: 11 g • C: 43 g • P: 359 mg • K: 1848 mg • Na: 932 mg

Cream of pumpkin

Preparation:

1. Peel and dice pumpkin and carrot.

2. Fry onion in olive oil.

3. Add pumpkin and carrots.

4. Fry for about 10 minutes.

5. Cook vegetable stock.

6. Pour broth over pumpkin and carrots.

7. Cook until vegetables are soft.

8. Add vanilla bean.

9. Blend to smooth cream.

10. Season with salt and pepper, garnish with pumpkin seeds.

SNACK

Proposition 1

Product	Kcal	Weight	Home measure
Strawberries	22	70 g	1 handful
Raspberries	31	60 g	1 handful
Blueberries	29	50 g	1 handful
Gelatin desserts dry mix	164	43 g	0.5 packaging
Natural yogurt 2%	12	20 g	1 tbsp

Kcal: 258 • P: 6 g • F: 1 g • C: 60 g • P: 125 mg • K: 279 mg • Na: 215 mg

Fruit in jelly

Preparation:

1. Prepare jelly according to the instructions on package.

2. Wash the fruits and pour over jelly. Put in refrigerator to let jelly set.

3. Add yogurt on top of dessert.

Proposition 2

Product	Kcal	Weight	Home measure
Coconut yogurt	75	80 g	0.5 packaging
Natural yogurt 2%	37	60 g	3 tbsp
Cocoa powder	11	5 g	1tsp
Blueberries	29	50 g	1 handful
Nectarine	48	110 g	small 1 piece
Raspberries	31	60 g	1 handful

Kcal: 231 • P: 7 g • F: 8 g • C: 38 g • P: 162 mg • K: 546 mg • Na: 46 mg

Yogurt with fruit

Preparation:

1. Mix yogurt with remaining ingredients.

Proposition 3

Product	Kcal	Weight	Home measure
Carrot	46	140 g	large 2 piece
Pear	107	160 g	small 1 piece
Lemon juice	1	6 g	1 tbsp
Walnuts	98	15 g	1 tbsp

Kcal: 253 • P: 4 g • F: 10 g • C: 40 g • P: 124 mg • K: 716 mg • Na: 99 mg

Carrot salad and nuts

Preparation:

1. Wash, peel and grate carrots on a coarse grater.

2. Dice peeled pear, sprinkle with lemon juice, add carrots and mix.

3. Sprinkle the top with chopped nuts.

Proposition 4

Product	Kcal	Weight	Home measure
Water	0	250 g	1 glass
Pineapple	50	110 g	1 serving
Lemon juice	7	30 g	5 tbsp
Ginger root	3	4 g	2 slice
Linseed	27	5 g	1tsp
Parsley leaves	9	24 g	2 tbsp
Biscuits	171	45 g	large 5 piece

Kcal: 265 • P: 7 g • F: 5 g • C: 52 g • P: 138 mg • K: 409 mg • Na: 88 mg

Smoothie with pineapple and parsley

Preparation:

1. Blend all ingredients, adding water as needed. 2. Eat biscuits.

Proposition 5

Product	Kcal	Weight	Home measure
Light rye bread	150	60 g	2 slice
Italian style cheese Capri (Sierpc)	75	40 g	4tsp
Avocado	24	15 g	1 slice
Lettuce butterhead	4	30 g	1 handful

Kcal: 253 • P: 8 g • F: 9 g • C: 38 g • P: 93 mg • K: 244 mg • Na: 444 mg

Capri cheese and lettuce sandwiches

Preparation:

1. Spread the sandwiches with capri cheese.

2. Add lettuce and sliced avocado.

Proposition 6

Product	Kcal	Weight	Home measure
Oat flakes	61	16 g	4tsp
Kiwi	46	75 g	1 piece
Strawberries	45	140 g	2 handful
Rice milk	94	200 g	200 ml
Cinnamon ground	10	4 g	1tsp

Kcal: 255 • P: 5 g • F: 4 g • C: 54 g • P: 239 mg • K: 577 mg • Na: 83 mg

Oat and rice smoothie

Preparation:

1. Pour boiling water over oatmeal, set aside for 3 minutes and blend with rest of ingredients.

2. If necessary, add water.

Proposition 7

Product	Kcal	Weight	Home measure
Hummus	142	60 g	3 tbsp
Light rye bread	150	60 g	2 slice
Radish sprouts	10	24 g	3 tbsp

Kcal: 305 • P: 8 g • F: 12 g • C: 44 g • P: 211 mg • K: 307 mg • Na: 619 mg

Sandwiches with hummus

Preparation:

1. Spread paste on the bread.

2. Decorate sandwiches with sprouts.

Proposition 8

Product	Kcal	Weight	Home measure
Coconut milk canned light 6%	80	120 g	0.5 glass
Coconut cream	61	10 g	1tsp
Avocado	112	70 g	0.5 piece
Orange	101	160 g	small 1 piece
Banana	89	100 g	small 1 piece
Ginger root	2	2 g	1tsp

Kcal: 444 • P: 7 g • F: 24 g • C: 57 g • P: 94 mg • K: 1281 mg • Na: 41 mg

Green smoothies

Preparation:

1. Blend the ingredients.

Proposition 9

Product	Kcal	Weight	Home measure
Apple	104	200 g	large 1 piece
Honey	36	12 g	1tsp
Walnuts	98	15 g	1 tbsp
Cinnamon ground	5	2 g	0.5 tsp

Kcal: 244 • P: 3 g • F: 10 g • C: 41 g • P: 76 mg • K: 295 mg • Na: 3 mg

Baked apple with cinnamon, nuts and honey

Preparation:

1. Bake apple in oven.

2. Add rest of ingredients.

DINNER

Proposition 1

Product	Kcal	Weight	Home measure
Butter	100	14 g	2tsp
Spinach	11	75 g	3 handful
Egg	70	50 g	medium 1 piece
Light rye bread	150	60 g	2 slice
Red tomato	31	170 g	1 piece
Pickled cucumber	14	130 g	medium 2 piece

Kcal: 376 • P: 12 g • F: 18 g • C: 46 g • P: 258 mg • K: 781 mg • Na: 2111 mg

Scrambled eggs with spinach

Preparation:

1. Heat half of butter in a pan, throw in spinach and blanch.

2. Whisk egg with salt and pepper in a separate dish. Pour into skillet.

3. Stir constantly until the egg is set.

4. Spread bread with butter and add tomato slices and pickled cucumber.

Proposition 2

Product	Kcal	Weight	Home measure
Corn pasta	179	50 g	50g
Avocado	112	70 g	0.5 piece
Lettuce butterhead	8	60 g	2 handful
Radish	5	30 g	2 piece
Mozzarella cheese	90	30 g	2 slice

Kcal: 393 • P: 13 g • F: 18 g • C: 49 g • P: 295 mg • K: 722 mg • Na: 167 mg

Salad with noodles and avocado

Preparation:

1. Cook pasta according to instructions on the package.

2. Chop vegetables and mozzarella.

3. Mix all ingredients.

4. Season.

Proposition 3

Product	Kcal	Weight	Home measure
White rice	210	60 g	4 tbsp
Apple	146	280 g	2 medium piece
Cinnamon ground	5	2 g	0.5 tsp
Coconut shreds	79	12 g	2 tbsp

Kcal: 440 • P: 6 g • F: 9 g • C: 90 g • P: 99 mg • K: 420 mg • Na: 12 mg

Rice with apple and coconut chips

Preparation:

1. Cook rice according to the instructions on the package. 2. Grate apple and combine whole thing, adding cinnamon.

3. Sprinkle whole thing with coconut shavings.

Proposition 4

Product	Kcal	Weight	Home measure
Beets cooked	106	240 g	2 piece
Arugula	4	20 g	1 handful
Ricotta cheese	90	60 g	3 tbsp
Lemon juice	3	12 g	2 tbsp
Olive oil	88	10 g	1 tbsp
Salt	0	1 g	1 pinch
Pepper black	5	2 g	2 pinch
Basil fresh	2	10 g	1 handful
Light rye bread	75	30 g	1 slice

Kcal: 373 • P: 11 g • F: 17 g • C: 49 g • P: 241 mg • K: 1056 mg • Na: 826 mg

Beet carpaccio on arugula and cottage cheese

Preparation:

1. Cut beets into thin slices.

2 Arrange a handful of arugula in the center of the plate, and overlap the beet slices all around. Add ricotta cheese.

3. Mix lemon juice well with olive oil, salt and pepper. Pour the dressing over the salad. Decorate whole thing with basil.

4. Serve with bread toasted in the toaster or oven.

Proposition 5

Product	Kcal	Weight	Home measure
Pepper red	16	60 g	medium 0.5 piece
Carrot	17	50 g	small 1 piece
Canola oil	177	20 g	2 tbsp
Parsley leaves	4	12 g	1 tbsp
White rice	175	50 g	0.5 package

Kcal: 388 • P: 5 g • F: 21 g • C: 48 g • P: 79 mg • K: 392 mg • Na: 47 mg

Vegetable salad with rice

Preparation:

1. Cut peppers and carrots into strips and fry in 1 tablespoon of oil.

2. Cook rice according to the instructions on the package.

3. Put vegetables in a bowl, add chopped parsley, rice, the rest of the oil and mix.

4. Season whole thing to taste.

Proposition 6

Product	Kcal	Weight	Home measure
Rice noodles	218	60 g	60g
Raspberries	62	120 g	2 handful
Natural yogurt 2%	37	60 g	3 tbsp
Honey	73	24 g	2tsp
Cinnamon ground	5	2 g	0.5 tsp

Kcal: 395 • P: 8 g • F: 2 g • C: 88 g • P: 202 mg • K: 340 mg • Na: 149 mg

Pasta with raspberry sauce

Preparation:

1. Cook pasta according to the instructions on the package.

2. Crush raspberries, add yogurt and honey, mix.

3. Pour sauce over pasta, sprinkle with cinnamon.

Proposition 7

Product	Kcal	Weight	Home measure
Avocado	112	70 g	0.5 piece
Lemon juice	1	6 g	1 tbsp
Olive oil	88	10 g	1 tbsp
Salt	0	1 g	1 pinch
Pepper black	3	1 g	1 pinch
Light rye bread	150	60 g	2 slice
Red tomato	11	60 g	medium 0.5 piece
Kiwi	46	75 g	1 piece

Kcal: 411 • P: 5 g • F: 22 g • C: 55 g • P: 153 mg • K: 835 mg • Na: 760 mg

Toast with avocado, kiwi

Preparation:

1. Mash avocado with a fork. Add lemon juice, olive oil, salt and pepper, mix.

2. Spread the bread slices with paste, add tomato slices.

3. Eat fruit separately.

Proposition 8

Product	Kcal	Weight	Home measure
Rye bread	91	35 g	1 slice
Vegan slices with pistachios (Go Vege)	13	12 g	1 slice
Royal cheese	53	15 g	1 slice
Mustard	10	10 g	1tsp
Sprouts mix	5	8 g	1 tbsp
Pickled cucumber	4	37 g	small 1 piece

Kcal: 176 • P: 8 g • F: 7 g • C: 21 g • P: 131 mg • K: 105 mg • Na: 1146 mg

Toast with ham and cheese

Preparation:

1. Toast bread in a toaster or toaster oven.

2. Brush toast with mustard, put vegan "ham", cheese and vegetables.

Proposition 9

Product	Kcal	Weight	Home measure
Wheat-rye bread	135	60 g	2 slice
Paste with grilled eggplant (Wawrzyniec)	58	40 g	2 tbsp

Kcal: 193 • P: 5 g • F: 8 g • C: 30 g • P: 77 mg • K: 216 mg • Na: 354 mg

Sandwich with eggplant paste

Preparation:

1. Spread the sandwich with vegetable paste.

Proposition 10

Product	Kcal	Weight	Home measure
Egg	140	100 g	2 medium piece
Milk 2%	23	45 g	3 tbsp
Oat flour	121	30 g	3 tbsp
Vanilla pudding without sugar	30	8 g	2tsp
Strawberries	45	140 g	2 handful

Kcal: 359 • P: 19 g • F: 14 g • C: 41 g • P: 406 mg • K: 529 mg • Na: 218 mg

Pudding omelette

Preparation:

1. Break the eggs, separate the whites from the yolks. Beat egg whites with a pinch of salt until stiff. In a bowl, mix egg yolks with milk, flour and pudding powder. Then add the egg whites in batches, mixing gently each time.

2. Pour the egg and pudding mixture into a non-fat frying pan, spread it evenly, reduce the heat and cook for a few minutes.

3. Slide the bottom-fried omelette onto a large plate, cover it with the pan and flip it over so that the un-fried side is on the bottom of the pan.

4. Fry for about 2 minutes.

5. Serve the omelette with fruit.

Read Nutrition Labels

Nutrition Facts

Serving Size 1 cup (110g)
Servings Per Container About 6

Amount Per Serving

Calories 250   Calories from Fat 30

% Daily Value*

Total Fat 7g	**11%**
Saturated Fat 3g	**16%**
Trans Fat 0g	
Cholesterol 4mg	**2%**
Sodium 300mg	**13%**
Total Carbohydrate 30g	**10%**
Dietary Fiber 3g	**14%**
Sugars 2g	
Protein 5g	

Vitamin A	7%
Vitamin C	15%
Calcium	20%
Iron	32%

* Percent Daily Values are based on a 2,000 calorie diet.
  Your daily value may be higher or lower depending on
  your calorie needs.

		Calories:	2,000	2,500
Total Fat	Less than		55g	75g
Saturated Fat	Less than		10g	12g
Cholesterol	Less than		1,500mg	1,700mg
Total Carbohydrate			250mg	300mg
Dietary Fiber			22mg	31mg

A   Serving size: This information is provided in familiar units that consumers use (1 cup, 15 cookies, etc.).

B   Servings per container: This indicates how many servings of food are in the container. Note: All nutrient values listed are for one
serving of food.

C   Calories: This is the number of calories in one serving of food.

D   Total fat: This is the total content of all fats—unhealthy and healthy—in one serving of food. Note: By law, food manufacturers are required to list only the unhealthy fat content in a food (saturated and trans fats), due to their role

in the development of cardiovascular disease.

Look for foods that have 2 grams or less of saturated or trans saturated fats per serving.

Healthy fats—monounsaturated and polyunsaturated fats (which are not required to be listed but still may be in the food item)—should be consumed in moderation.

Choose foods that have less than 3 grams of total fat per serving, which is considered low-fat.

Some nutrient claims on labels can also be useful in selecting heart-healthy food items. Look for claims like "saturated fat-free," "sodium-free," "low saturated fat," and "no trans fat."

E   Sodium: As mentioned, the recommended daily intake of sodium is limited to about 2,000 milligrams. The Food and Drug Administration mandates that milligrams of sodium per serving must be listed for all food items. This takes the

serving.

High-sodium foods: Avoid foods containing more than 500 milligrams per serving.

Nutrient claims on labels can also help guide your food selections. Look for "very low sodium," "low sodium," and "reduced salt." Foods must meet certain requirements to use these claims.

Phosphorus: Most CKD patients are limited to between 800 and 1,000 milligrams of phosphorus per day (your specific needs can be determined by your health care team). Phosphorus content is not required by law to be listed on the nutrient facts label, but here's a trick to get that information from the ingredients list. To determine if a food product has had phosphorus added, look for any ingredient that contains the four letters "phos." Phosphorus is naturally occurring in animal and plant protein sources, so foods that have added phosphorus should be avoided completely. If phosphorus additives are on the ingredient list, do yourself a favor and put that food product back on the shelf.

Phosphorus additives include the following:

Phos phoric acid

Sodium poly phos phate

Pyro phos phate

Sodium tripoly phos phate

Poly phos phate

Tricalcium phos phate

Hexameta phos phate

Trisodium phos phate

Dicalcium phos phate

Sodium phos phate

Tetrasodium phos phate

Aluminum phos phate Potassium: Most CKD patients are limited to about 2,000 milligrams of
potassium per day (your specific needs can be determined by your health care team). Potassium is another nutrient that is not required by law to be listed on the nutrient facts label, but you can get some helpful information by reading the ingredients list. Potassium is naturally occurring in many fruits, vegetables, and dairy products, but it can also be added for flavor and as a preservative to many processed

Steer clear of food items that have any potassium additives, such as the following:

Potassium acetates

Potassium alginate

Potassium alum

Potassium bisulfite

Potassium bromate

Potassium carbonate

Potassium caseinate

Potassium chloride

Potassium citrates

Potassium gluconate

Potassium hydroxide

Potassium nitrate

Potassium phosphates

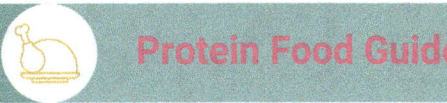

Protein Food Guide

High-protein food sources
(10 grams or more of protein per serving)

Food	Serving size	Grams of protein
Meat		
Beef, ground, 80% lean	3 ounce	20
Beef, ground, 97% lean	3 ounce	22
Beef (top round, bottom	3 ounce	24-26
round) Beef, roast beef	3 ounce	23
Chicken, breast	3.5 ounce (½ breast)	29
Chicken (white, dark)	3 ounce	20-22
Fish (fried)	3 ounce	15
Lamb (leg)	3 ounce	22
Sardines, with bone	1 can (3.75 ounce)	23
Pork, tenderloin	3 ounce	22
Crab	3 ounce	15
Crab, Alaska	1 leg	22
Tuna (light, in water)	3 ounce	21.7
Turkey, (white, dark)	3 ounce	24-26
Clams, fried	20 small	27
Cod, Atlantic	3 ounce	19
Haddock	1 fillet	30
Salmon, fresh	3 ounce	19
Pollock	3 ounce	21
Shrimp	3 ounce	20
Dairy		
Cheese, cottage (1% milkfat)	4 ounce	14
Cheese, mozzarella	½ cup	12
Plant/Grains		
Veggie/soy patty	1 patty	11
Spaghetti	1 cup	13

Medium-protein food sources
(4–9 grams or more of protein per serving)

Food	Serving size	Grams of protein
Meat/Eggs		
Egg, substitute	¼ cup	6 6
Egg, whole, large	1 large	6
Hot dog	1 (hot dog)	6-8
Meat, deli sliced (ham, turkey, chicken)	3 slices	
Dairy		
Cheese, American	1 ounce	5 4
Ice cream, vanilla soft serve	½ cup	4
Milk, 2%	½ cup	9
Milk, evaporated, canned	½ cup	4.5
Pudding, prepared with milk	½ cup	6
Yogurt, plain, whole milk	1 container (6 ounce)	
Plant/Grains		
Beans, kidney (canned)	½ cup	7
Beans, baked (canned)	½ cup	6
Lentils	½ cup	9
Peas	½ cup	4
Nuts, cashews, walnuts, mixed	1 ounce	4
Nuts, peanuts, pistachios, almonds	1 ounce	6
Seeds, sunflower	1 ounce	5
Seeds, pumpkin	1 ounce	8
Soybeans (edamame)	½ cup	9
Soy, milk	1 cup	6
Tofu, firm	¼ cup	9
Peanut butter, chunky	2 tbsp	8
Bagel	1 small bagel (3½ inch diameter)	7
Roll, hamburger or hotdog	1 roll	4
Muffin, English	1 muffin	4
Cereal, granola	½ cup	6

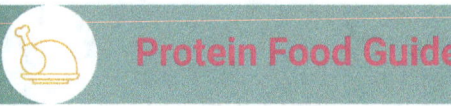
Low-protein food sources
(Less than 4 grams of protein per serving)

Food	Serving size	Grams of protein
Dairy		
Cheese, parmesan	2 tablespoon	3
Cheese, cream	1 tablespoon	1
Cream, light or half & half (fat free)	2 tablespoon	1
Sour cream	½ cup	3
Yogurt, frozen, vanilla	½ cup	3
Plant/Grains		
Beans, green/yellow snap	½ cup	1
Beets, canned	½ cup slices	1
Bread, pita	1 each (large 6 ½ inch)	5
Bread, white wheat	1 slice	3
Broccoli, cooked	½ cup, chopped	2
Brussels sprouts	½ cup	1
Cauliflower, chopped ½ pieces	½ cup	1

Food	Serving size	Grams of protein
Cereal, raisin bran	1 cup	4
Corn, kernel	½ cup	2
Cream of wheat	1 cup	4
Collard Greens	½ cup	3
Muffin, Blueberry	1 small	3
Mushrooms, canned	½ cup	1
Oatmeal, dry	⅓ cup	4
Pancake (4-inch)	1 each	2
Peas, green, canned	½ cup	4
Potato, baked with skin	1 medium	4
Rice, brown	½ cup	3
Rice, wild	½ cup	3
Spinach, cooked	½ cup	3
Tomato sauce	½ cup	2
Tortilla, flour	1 tortilla	4

Potassium Food Guide

Protein

Low potassium 150 mg or less per serving		
Meat	**Serving size**	**Potassium (mg)**
Ground beef,	3 oz	135
lean Roast beef	3 oz	150
Nuts		
Brazilnut	1 oz (1 nut)	33
Pecans	1 oz (20 halves)	116
Walnuts	1 oz (14 halves)	12
Seafood		5
Oysters, raw	6	131

Medium potassium 151-250 mg per serving		
Beans, canned	**Serving size**	**Potassium (mg)**
Blackeyed	½ cup	207
Garbanzo/Chickpea	½ cup	207
Meat		
Chicken breast, no skin	3 oz	220
Nuts		
Almonds	1 oz (24 nuts)	201
Cashews	1 oz (18 nuts)	160
Coconut, sweet	½ cup	157
Macadamia	1 oz (10–12 nuts)	103
Peanut butter	2 tbsp	230
Seeds		
Pumpkin	1 oz	229
Sunflower	1 oz	241
Seafood		
Catfish, breaded	3 oz	289
Crab, Alaskan	3 oz	223
Shrimp	3 oz	155
Tuna, canned	3 oz	200

High potassium 251 mg or more per serving		
Beans	**Serving size**	**Potassium (mg)**
Baked	½ cup	376
Beans, canned		
Black	½ cup	305
Great Northern	½ cup	460
Kidney	½ cup	304
Lentils	½ cup	365
Lima	½ cup	265
Navy	½ cup	587
*Refried	½ cup	535
Pinto	½ cup	292
*Soybeans	½ cup	443
Meat		
Ham	3 oz	300
Lamb	3 oz	265
*Pork loin/chop	3 oz	370
Turkey, light/dark	3 oz	251
*Veal, roasted	3 oz	251
Nuts		
Pistachio	1 oz	295
Seafood		
Clams, raw	3 oz	267
*Cod	3 oz	440
*Haddock	3 oz	339
Lobster	3 oz	300
Pollock	3 oz	329
*Salmon, fresh	3 oz	319
Scallops	6 large	300
*Tuna, fresh	3 oz	484

* = 200 mg of **phosphorus** or greater

>

Potassium Food Guide

Milk & Dairy

Low potassium
150 mg or less per serving

Cheese	Serving size	Potassium (mg)
*American	1 oz	6
Blue	1 oz	9
Cheddar	1 oz	71
Cottage	½ cup	28
Cream	1 oz	97
Feta	1 oz	17
Mozzarella	1 oz	17
Parmesan	2 tbsp	27
Swiss	1 oz	12
Cream		31
Heav	1	11
y	tbsp	17
Eggs	1	
Egg, whole, fresh	tbsp 1.5 oz	70
Ice cream		
Vanilla	½ cup	131
Pudding cup		
Vanilla	4 oz	128

Medium potassium
151-250 mg per serving

Cheese	Serving size	Potassium (mg)
*Ricotta (part skim)	½ cup	153
Eggs		
Egg substitute	¼ cup	207
Ice cream		
Chocolate	½ cup	164

Medium potassium, cont.

Milk	Serving size	Potassium (mg)
Buttermilk	½ cup	185
Chocolate	½ cup	210
Skim	½ cup	204
1% low fat	½ cup	190
Whole	½ cup	185
Soy	½ cup	173
Pudding, instant		
Chocolate	½ cup	215
Vanilla	½ cup	190
Pudding cup		
Chocolate	4 oz	201
Yogurt		
Frozen yogurt	½ cup	152

High potassium
251 mg or more per serving

Milk	Serving size	Potassium (mg)
Condensed	½ cup	567
*Evaporated	½ cup	425
Yogurt		
Yogurt, plain, low fat	4 oz	266

* = 200 mg of **phosphorus** or greater

>

Potassium Food Guide

Fruit & Fruit Juices

Low potassium 150 mg or less per serving		
Fruits	**Serving size**	**Potassium (mg)**
Applesauce	½ cup	78
Apricot, raw	1	104
Blackberries, raw	½ cup	141
Blueberries, raw	½ cup	65
Grapes	10 grapes	93
Lemon	1 medium sized	80
Mango	½ cup	128
Pears, canned	½ cup	119
Pineapple, raw	½ cup	88
Plum	1 medium sized	114
Raspberries, raw	½ cup	94
Rhubarb, cooked, sweetened	½ cup	115
Strawberries, raw	½ cup	138
Tangerine oranges, raw	1 small	132
Juices		
Apple	½ cup	148
Cranberry	½ cup	23
Grape	½ cup	26
Apricot nectar	½ cup	143
Peach nectar	½ cup	50
Pear nectar	½ cup	16

Medium potassium 151-250 mg per serving		
Fruits	**Serving size**	**Potassium (mg)**
Apple, raw	½ cup	159
Apricots, canned	½ cup	200
Cherries	10 cherries	152
Fruit cocktail	½ cup	210
Grapefruit	1 half	159
Guava, raw	½ cup	235

Medium potassium, cont.		
Fruits	**Serving size**	**Potassium (mg)**
Cantaloupe	½ cup	247
Honeydew	½ cup	230
Orange	1 medium sized	237
Papaya	½ cup	180
Peaches, canned/raw	½ cup	160
Pear	1 medium sized	208
Pineapple, canned	½ cup	152
Plums, canned	½ cup	194
Watermelon	½ cup	176
Juices		
Grapefruit	½ cup	203
Orange	½ cup	237
Pineapple	½ cup	168

High potassium 251 mg or more per serving		
Fruits	**Serving size**	**Potassium (mg)**
Banana	1 medium sized	467
Dates	½ cup	581
Figs, dried	2	271
Kiwi	1 medium sized	252
Nectarines	1 medium sized	288
Passion fruit, purple	½ cup	410
Persimmon, Japanese	½ cup	270
Plantain, cooked	½ cup	360
Pomegranate	1 medium sized	399
Prunes, dried	½ cup	415
Raisins	½ cup	545
Juices		
Prune	½ cup	354
Passion fruit juice, purple/yellow	½ cup	344

* = 200 mg of **phosphorus** or greater

Vegetables

Low potassium
150 mg or less per serving

Vegetables	Serving size	Potassium (mg)
Beans, green/yellow	½ cup	85
Beets, canned	½ cup	126
Broccoli, raw	½ cup	139
Cabbage, green, raw	½ cup	86
Carrots, canned	½ cup	131
Cauliflower, cooked	½ cup	115
Corn, frozen, kernel	½ cup	121
Cucumber, with peel	½ cup	75
Eggplant, cooked	½ cup	123
Lettuce	½ cup	43
Mushrooms, raw	½ cup	130
Mustard greens, cooked Onion, raw	½ cup	141
	½ cup	126
Peas, canned	½ cup	148
Peppers, green	½ cup	132
Radishes, raw	½ cup	135
Spinach, raw	½ cup	84
Turnips, cooked	½ cup	106
Turnip greens, cooked	½ cup	146

Medium potassium
151-250 mg per serving

Vegetables	Serving size	Potassium (mg)
Asparagus, canned/frozen	½ cup	200
Broccoli, cooked	½ cup	228
Brussels sprouts, cooked	½ cup	250
Carrots, raw	½ cup	178
Celery, raw	½ cup	172
Collards, cooked	½ cup	246
Corn, creamed	½ cup	171
Sauerkraut, canned	½ cup	201
Squash, summer, cooked	½ cup	173
Tomato, fresh, raw	½ cup	200

High potassium
251 mg or more per serving

Vegetables	Serving size	Potassium (mg)
Artichoke	1 medium sized	425
Avocado	½ cup	558
Bamboo shoots canned	½ cup	533
Beet greens	½ cup	650
Cabbage, Chinese, cooked	½ cup	315
Kohlrabi, cooked	½ cup	280
Okra, cooked	½ cup	258
Parsnips	½ cup	286
Pumpkin, canned	½ cup	253
Rutabagas, cooked	½ cup	277
Spinach, cooked	½ cup	420
Squash, winter, cooked	½ cup	448
Vegetable juice	½ cup	234

Potatoes

Vegetables	Serving size	Potassium (mg)
Au gratin	½ cup	485
Baked	1 medium sized	610
Boiled	1 medium sized	515
French fried	½ cup	550
Hash browned	½ cup	251
Mashed	½ cup	315
Scalloped	½ cup	463
Sweet	1 medium sized	855
Yams (sweet potato), canned	½ cup	398

Tomatoes

Vegetables	Serving size	Potassium (mg)
Juice	½ cup	267
Paste	½ cup	1228
Sauce	½ cup	454
Whole	½ cup	265

* = 200 mg of **phosphorus** or greater

Potassium Food Guide

Cereals & Starches

Low potassium (mg) 150 mg or less per serving		
Cereal	**Serving size**	**Potassium (mg)**
Cheerios™	1 cup	96
Corn Flakes*	1 cup	22
Rice Krispies*	1 cup	35
Hot cereals		
Cream of	1 cup	48
Wheat* Grits	1 cup	51
Malt-o-meal*	1 cup	31
Oatmeal	1 cup	131
Muffins		
Banana	small	65
*Blueberry	small	70
Wheat bran	small	60
Starches		
Bagel	3 ½" plain	72
Biscuit	1-4" plain	122
Bread	1 slice, white/ wheat	50
Cornbread	2" square	96
Crackers	4 squares	15
Croissant	small	67
Pancake, buttermilk	2 small	110
Pasta	½ cup, cooked	45
Rice, white	½ cup, cooked	33
Roll, dinner	small	40
Tortilla, corn or flour	1	41
Waffles		
Homemade	1	120
Frozen	1	42

Medium potassium (mg) 151-250 mg per serving		
Cereal	**Serving size**	**Potassium (mg)**
Complete Bran Flakes	1 cup	228
Frosted Mini Wheats*	1 cup	190
Muffin		
*Oat bran	small	289

High potassium (mg) 251 mg or more per serving		
Cereal	**Serving size**	**Potassium (mg)**
Raisin Bran	1 cup	372
All Bran	1 cup	678
Granola, w/raisins	1 cup	420
Starches		
Pancakes, wheat	2 small	251

* = 200 mg of phosphorus or greater

 Remember: Potassium values depend on portion sizes. Foods low in potassium can become high potassium foods if a larger portion is eaten.

Potassium Food Guide

Beverages, Sweets, and Processed Foods

Low potassium
150 mg or less per serving

Beverages, alcoholic	Serving size	Potassium (mg)
Beer	12 fl oz	89
Coffee	1 cup	128
Red wine	3.5oz	115
White wine	3.5 oz	82
Beverages, non-alcoholic		
Cola	12 fl oz	4
Lemon/lime soda	12 fl oz	4
Orange soda	12 fl oz	7
Tea	1 cup	88
Cake		
Angel food	1" slice	26
Chocolate	2 x 2" slice	126
White	2 x 2" slice	70
Condiments		
Ketchup	2 tbsp	144
Cookies		
Chocolate chip	1 each	36
Fig bar	1 each	33
Grahams	2 squares	19
Oatmeal raisin	1 each	36
Peanut butter	1 each	46
Sugar	1 each	11
Vanilla wafer	1 each	4
Gelatin		
Gelatin	½ cup	1
Pie		
Apple	⅛ pie	122
Cherry	⅛ pie	139

Low potassium, cont.

Snacks	Serving size	Potassium (mg)
Popcorn	1 cup	25
Pretzels	10 each	88
Tortilla chips, plain, nacho cheese		60
Sherbet		
Orange	½ cup	71
Soup (made w/water)		
Beef noodle	1 cup	100
Chicken noodle	1 cup	108
Cream of chicken	1 cup	88
Cream of mushroom	1 cup	100

Medium potassium
151-250 mg per serving

Beverages	Serving size	Potassium(mg)
Cocoa mix (made with water)	1 cup	202
Eggnog	½ cup	210
Pie		
Pecan	⅛ pie	162
Snacks		
Chocolate bar	1.5 oz	169
Soup (made w/water)		
Split pea	1 cup	190
Vegetable beef	1 cup	173

>

Potassium Food Guide

Beverages, Sweets, and Processed Foods, cont.

High potassium		
251 mg or more per serving		
Beverages	**Serving size**	**Potassium (mg)**
*Cocoa mix, sugar-free, (made w/milk)	1 cup	405
Condiments		
Salt substitute	¼ tsp	800
Meat		
Cheeseburger, plain	1	360
Chili (w/ beans)	1 cup	691
Taco	small	474
Pie		
Pumpkin	⅛ pie	288

Potato chips	Serving size	Potassium (mg)
BBQ	1 oz bag	357
Plain	1 oz bag	361
Low fat	1 oz bag	491
Snacks		
*Trail mix	½ cup	495
Soup (made w/water)		
Chicken vegetable	1 cup	367
Clam chowder	1 cup	300
Minestrone	1 cup	313
Tomato	1 cup	264

= 200 mg of **phosphoru** or greater

Estimate Portion Sizes Using Your Hand

This portion size guide can help you identify how much is on the plate without having to measure out your portions. For example, if what is on the plate looks as if it is double the size of a palm, then the serving size of 3 oz is doubled.

The Palm = 3 oz.

The palm of your hand can be used to estimate protein intake. 1 palm is equivalent to a 3 oz. serving of protein. Examples of what you could measure a 3 oz. serving include pork, poultry, beef, fish, and chicken.

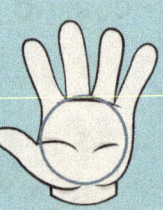

Fist = 1 cup

A fist is a great way of measuring carbohydrates. You can use this tool when measuring the intake of rice, cereals, salads, fruits, or popcorn.

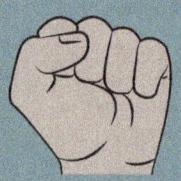

Tip of Thumb = 1 Tablespoon

The tip of a thumb is equivalent to a serving of 1 tablespoon. This tool is used when measuring fat intake such as mayonnaise, cheese, salad dressings, creams, and peanut butter.

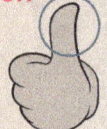

A Cupped Hand = 1/2 cup

1 hand cupped is equivalent to a 1/2 cup serving. You can use this tool for measuring food items such as pastas, potatoes, nuts, and even ice cream.

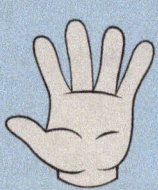

The Thumb Nail – 1 Teaspoon

The nail of the thumb is about 1 teaspoon serving of oils or fats. This can be used to measure salad dressings, olive oil, or butter.

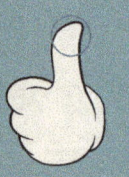

Other At Home Ways of Measuring:

There are many other resources you can use to measure aside from your hand or an actual measuring cup.

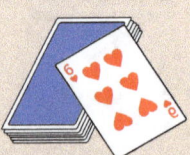

A deck of cards = 3 oz serving of protein

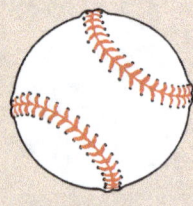

A softball = 2 cups

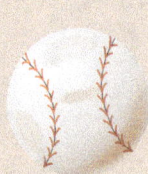

A baseball = 1 cup

A tennis ball = 1/2 cup

A golf ball = 2 tablespoons

Note about measurements:

US Customary cup = 236ml is defined as 8 oz or 1/2 pint and was used customarily throughout United States. But it seems this is no longer popular. US Metric cup = 250ml is what you will find in most stores. Betty Crocker defines 1 cup as 250 ml. Therefore, this book uses the metric of 1 cup = 250ml.

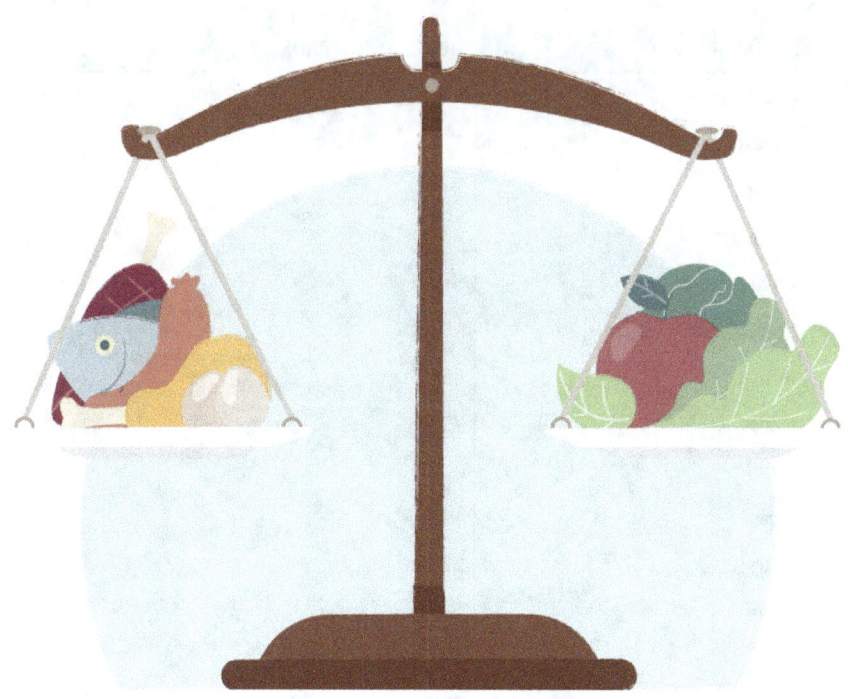

Measurements and Conversions

Volume Equivalents (Dry)

US STANDARD	METRIC (APPROX.)
⅛ teaspoon	0.5 mL
¼ teaspoon	1 mL
½ teaspoon	2 mL
¾ teaspoon	4 mL
1 teaspoon	5 mL
1 tablespoon	15 mL
¼ cup	59 mL
⅓ cup	79 mL
½ cup	118 mL
⅔ cup	156 mL
¾ cup	177 mL
1 cup	235 mL
2 cups or 1 pint	475 mL
3 cups	700 mL

4 cups or 1 quart ½ gallon	1 L
quart ½ gallon	2 L
1 gallon	4 L

Volume Equivalents (Liquid)

US STANDARD	US STANDARD (OUNCES)	METRIC (APPROX.)
2 tablespoons	1 fl. oz.	30 mL
¼ cup	2 fl. oz.	60 mL
½ cup	4 fl. oz.	120 mL
1 cup	8 fl. oz.	240 mL
1½ cups	12 fl. oz.	355 mL
2 cups or 1 pint	16 fl. oz.	475 mL
4 cups or 1 quart	32 fl. oz.	1 L
1 gallon	128 fl. oz.	4 L

Oven Temperatures

FAHRENHEIT (F)	CELSIUS (C) (APPROX.)
250°F	120°C
300°F	150°C
325°F	165°C
350°F	180°C
375°F	190°C
400°F	200°C
425°F	220°C
450°F	230°C

Weight Equivalents

US STANDARD	METRIC (APPROX.)
½ ounce	15 g
1 ounce	30 g
2 ounces	60 g
4 ounces	115 g
8 ounces	225 g
12 ounces	340 g
16 ounces or 1 pound	455 g

About the Author

Dr Barbara Pyszczuk

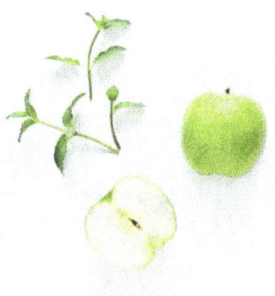

A graduate of the Faculty of Human Nutrition and Consumption Sciences at the Warsaw University of Life Sciences. Speaker at national and international scientific conferences. Author of numerous scientific and popular science publications in the field of nutrition. She cooperates daily, with patients with kidney diseases.

Published books and E-books.

Title:

1. A walk through the diet in urolithiasis. e - book and book

2. Low-protein diet in CKD. e - book

3. Gout – Dietotherapy. e - book

4. CKD tables.e - book

5. With Dialysis in the Land of Tastes. e - book and book

6. Diet in Kidney Disease Before Dialysis. e - book

7. 7-Day Kidney Disease Meal Plan and Recipes. e - book

8. 7 – Day Meal Plan For Dialysis Patients. e - book

www.doktorbarbara.pl
https://www.facebook.com/doktorbarbara/

www.ingramcontent.com/pod-product-compliance
Lightning Source LLC
Chambersburg PA
CBHW071100290526
45795CB00004B/1588